T0138565

MEDICAL APHORISMS

TREATISES 10–15

◆

NEAL A. MAXWELL INSTITUTE
FOR RELIGIOUS SCHOLARSHIP

MIDDLE EASTERN TEXTS INITIATIVE

EDITOR IN CHIEF
Daniel C. Peterson

MANAGING EDITOR
D. Morgan Davis

ASSOCIATE EDITOR
Muḥammad Eissa

VOLUME EDITOR
Angela C. Barrionuevo

◆

THE MEDICAL WORKS OF MOSES MAIMONIDES
ACADEMIC BOARD
Gerrit Bos (University of Cologne), *general editor*
Lawrence I. Conrad (University of Hamburg)
Alfred L. Ivry (New York University)
Y. Tzvi Langermann (Bar Ilan University, Israel)
Michael R. McVaugh (University of North Carolina, Chapel Hill)

◆

*This publication was funded through the support
of the U.S. Congress and the Library of Congress*

Maimonides

Medical Aphorisms
Treatises 10–15

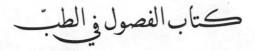

A parallel Arabic-English edition
edited, translated, and annotated by

Gerrit Bos

◆ ◆ ◆

PART OF THE MEDICAL WORKS

OF MOSES MAIMONIDES

Brigham Young University Press ◆ *Provo, Utah* ◆ *2010*

©2010 by Brigham Young University Press. All rights reserved.

Library of Congress Cataloging-in-Publication Data is available.

ISBN: 978–0–8425–2780–4 (alk. paper)

PRINTED IN THE UNITED STATES OF AMERICA.

1 2 3 4 5 6 7   16 15 14 13 12 11 10

First Edition

Contents

❖ ❖ ❖

Kitāb al fuṣūl fī al-ṭibb (Medical Aphorisms)

❖ ❖ ❖

Bibliographies

Sigla and Abbreviations

Arabic Manuscripts of the *Kitāb al-fuṣūl fī al-ṭibb*

G Gotha, orient. 1937, fols. 6–273.

L Leiden, Bibliotheek der Rijksuniversiteit 1344, Or. 128.1, fols. 1–140.

E Escorial, Real Biblioteca de El Escorial 868, fols. 117–26.

S Escorial, Real Biblioteca de El Escorial 869, fols. 176–1.

B Oxford, Bodleian, Uri 412, Poc. 319, cat. Neubauer 2113.

O Oxford, Bodleian, Hunt. Donat 33, Uri 423, cat. Neubauer 2114.

U Oxford, Bodleian, Hunt. 356, Uri 426, cat. Neubauer 2115.

Arabic Manuscripts of Galenic Works

A Ayasofya 3593, fols. 48a–51b, Galen, *Fī sū᾽ al-mizāj al-mukhtalif* (*De inaequali intemperie liber*), forthcoming edition by Gerrit Bos, Michael R. McVaugh, and Joseph Shatzmiller.

C Cairo, *Ṭal᾽at ṭibb* 550, *Tafsīr Jālīnūs li-kitāb Buqrāṭ fī al-ahwiya wa-al-buldān*. Arabic translation of Galen, *In Hippocratis De aere aquis locis commentarius*, forthcoming edition by G. Strohmaier.

H Paris, Bibliothèque nationale, arab. 2853, Galen, *Kitāb fī manāfiᶜ al-aᶜḍāᶜ* (De usu partium), Arabic translation by Ḥubaysh, revised by Ḥunayn.

W London, Wellcome Or. 14a, Galen, *Kitāb al-mawāḍiᶜ al-ālima* (De locis affectis), Arabic translation by Ḥunayn.

Hebrew Translations

N Hebrew translation by Nathan ha-Meᵓati, as found in Paris, Bibliothèque nationale, héb. 1173, *Sefer ha-Peraḳim.*

Z   Hebrew translation by Zeraḥyah ben Isaac ben Sheʾaltiel
            Ḥen, as found in Munich, Bayerische Staatsbibliothek 111,
            Sefer ha-Perakim.

A superscripted 1 after a siglum (e.g. G^1) indicates a note in the margin
of that manuscript. A superscripted 2 indicates a note above the line.

Other

Bo   Maimonides, *Aphorismi secundam doctrinam Galeni,* Latin trans-
            lation by Giovanni da Capua, ed. Bologna 1489.

m   Maimonides, *Pirḳe Mosheh bi-refuʾah,* Hebrew translation by
            Nathan ha-Meʾati, ed. Muntner.

r   Maimonides, *Medical Aphorisms,* English translation by Rosner.

Deller   Deichgräber and Deller, "Die Exzerpte des Moses Maimonides
            aus den Epidemienkommentaren des Galen."

◆ ◆ ◆

< >   supplied by editor, in Arabic text
[ ]   supplied by translator, in English text
(!)   corrupt reading
(?)   doubtful reading
add.   added in
emend. Bos conjecture or correction
om.   omitted in

Transliteration and Citation Style

Transliterations from Arabic and Hebrew follow the romanization tables
established by the American Library Association and the Library of Congress (*ALA-LC Romanization Tables: Transliteration Schemes for Non-Roman
Scripts.* Compiled and edited by Randall K. Barry. Washington, D.C.:
Library of Congress, 1997; available online at www.loc.gov/catdir/cpso/
roman.html).

Passages from *Medical Aphorisms* are referenced by treatise and section
number (e.g., 3.12). Maimonides' introduction is designated as treatise 0.

Foreword

Brigham Young University and its Middle Eastern Texts Initiative are pleased to sponsor and publish the Medical Works of Moses Maimonides. The texts that appear in this series are among the cultural treasures of the world, representing as they do the medieval efflorescence of Arabic-Islamic civilization—a civilization in which works of impressive intellectual stature were composed not only by Muslims but also by Christians, Jews, and others in a quest for knowledge that transcended religious and ethnic boundaries. Together they not only preserved the best of Greek thought but enhanced it, added to it, and built upon it a corpus of scientific and philosophical understanding that is properly the inheritance of all the peoples of the world.

As an institution of The Church of Jesus Christ of Latter-day Saints, Brigham Young University is honored to collaborate with Gerrit Bos and other members of the academic community in bringing this series to fruition, making these texts available to many for the first time. In doing so, we at the Middle Eastern Texts Initiative hope to serve our fellow human beings of all creeds and cultures. We also follow the admonition of our own religious tradition, to "seek . . . out of the best books words of wisdom," believing, indeed, that "the glory of God is intelligence."

—Daniel C. Peterson
—D. Morgan Davis

Preface

This edition of Maimonides' *Medical Aphorisms: Treatises 10–15* is the third volume in a series of five volumes that will cover all twenty-five treatises. In addition to these five volumes, a sixth volume, containing an extensive glossary of approximately 5000 terms of the Arabic text and the two Hebrew translations (by Nathan ha-Meʾati and Zeraḥyah ben Isaac ben Sheʾaltiel Ḥen) with alphabetical Hebrew indexes, is in preparation. Once completed, it will be added to the other glossaries that have been put on the internet to be consulted by the scholarly community. (See www.uni-koeln.de/phil-fak/juda/forschung/forschungsprojekte/maimonides/glossare.htm.)

This new edition is part of an ongoing project to critically edit Maimonides' medical works that have not been edited at all or have been edited in unreliable editions. This project started in 1995 at the University College London, with the support of the Wellcome Trust, and now is proceeding at the Martin Buber Institute for Jewish Studies at the University of Cologne with the financial support of the Deutsche Forschungsgemeinschaft. So far it has resulted in the publication of critical editions of Maimonides' *On Asthma* (2 vols.), *Medical Aphorisms* 1–9 (2 vols.), and *On Poisons*.

The series is published by the Middle Eastern Texts Initiative at Brigham Young University's Neal A. Maxwell Institute for Religious Scholarship. On this occasion I thank Professor Daniel C. Peterson, under whose direction this series has been prepared for publication, and his colleague, Dr. D. Morgan Davis, for their enthusiastic support of the project and dedication to it. I thank Professor Vivian Nutton for his help in identifying some Galenic sources. Thanks are also due to Angela C. Barrionuevo, Elizabeth Watkins, Jude Ogzewalla, and Muhammad S. Eissa for their diligent editorial work.

Translator's Introduction

This third volume of the critical edition of Maimonides'[1] *Medical Aphorisms* covers treatises 10–15. The central subjects of these treatises are fevers (treatise 10), periods and crisis of a disease (treatise 11), evacuation through bleeding (treatise 12), evacuation through purgatives and enemas (treatise 13), vomiting (treatise 14), and surgery (treatise 15). The interest such subjects aroused in Jewish circles is attested from an anonymous compilation on fevers, written in old French in Hebrew script and probably dating from the thirteenth century, in which the author remarks that he wants to translate everything from the "Pirkei Rabbenu Mosheh" concerning the "crisis [of fevers]."[2] And in his treatise on fevers, Salmias (Salamias) of Lunel quotes, in the name of Maimonides, a recipe for quartan fever found in aphorism 10.56 and derived from Galen's *De theriaca ad Pisonem*.[3]

Most of the aphorisms are based on the works of Galen, but Maimonides also cites other ancient and medieval physicians. Thus, he quotes a certain Asklepios, who wrote a now-lost commentary on Hippocrates' treatise *On Fractures*: "[Broken] bones of young people heal sooner than those of children, because children need material for their growth to replace the matter which has been dissolved. This was mentioned by

---

1. See the introduction to *On Poisons* for Maimonides' biographical and bibliographical data; see as well the recently published monumental monograph by Joel Kraemer: *Maimonides: The Life and World of One of Civilization's Greatest Minds*.

2. See Steinschneider, *Verzeichniss der hebräischen Handschriften,* no. 233; idem, "Eine altfranzösische Compilation," 401; cf. translator's introduction to the first volume of Maimonides, *Medical Aphorisms,* ed. and trans. Bos.

3. Cf. aphorism 10.56 in this volume. Salmias quotes from the Hebrew translation composed by Nathan ha-Meʾati. For other quotations attesting to the interest Maimonides' *Aphorisms* excited in Jewish circles, see the introductions to vols. 1 and 2.

Asklepios in the first treatise of his commentary on [Hippocrates'] book on [fractures] and their setting. Do not attempt to set any broken bone if only four days have passed, lest you cause the patient severe harm. The third [treatise] of Asklepios' commentary on [Hippocrates'] book on [fractures] and their setting" (aphorisms 15.63–64).

This commentary is unknown from bibliographical literature. Leclerc remarks that al-Rāzī, in his *Kitāb al-ḥāwī*, quotes a commentator to Hippocrates' *On Fractures* called Senflious, and that the Latin translator has rendered this name Herilius or Sterilius. He adds that this could be read as Simplicius.[4] Steinschneider[5] notes that سينبليقيوس (Sinblikius) is indeed the first commentator on Hippocrates mentioned by Ibn al-Nadīm in his *Kitāb al-fihrist*,[6] but adds that this name does not feature in the list of commentators found in Littré.[7] Ullmann identifies سنبلقيوس, i.e., the name of the commentator mentioned in al-Rāzī's *Kitāb al-ḥāwī*,[8] as Simplikios, and adds that he is otherwise unknown.[9] However, it seems more probable that the name of al-Rāzī's commentator is a corruption of اسقليبوس (*ᶜsqlbyws*)—i.e., Asklepios—and that he refers to the same Asklepios as Maimonides.

Other quotations, called "Rules in hortatory form" (*waṣāyā*), probably hail from a lost work entitled *Waṣīya* that was composed by Abū al-ᶜAlāʾ ibn Zuhr (d. 1131)[10] for his son Abū Marwān (d. 1162).[11] The central subject of these rules is the treatment by means of purgatives.[12] Maimonides' comment on one of these rules give us a fine insight into both his critical attitude and his experience as a physician. For when Abū al-ᶜAlāʾ remarks, "It is a mistake to use musk as part of purgatives,

---

4. Leclerc, *Histoire de la médecine arabe,* 1:235, 267; cf. Steinschneider, *Arabischen Übersetzungen aus dem Griechischen,* 308.

5. Steinschneider, *Arabischen Übersetzungen aus dem Griechischen,* 308.

6. Ibn al-Nadīm, *Kitāb al-fihrist,* 415 (ed. Flügel, 288).

7. Littré, *Oeuvres complètes d'Hippocrate,* 1:81–132.

8. al-Rāzī, *Kitāb al-ḥāwī fī al-ṭibb,* 13:159; the name actually found in this book is سنقليوس.

9. Ullmann, *Medizin im Islam,* 31, no. 12.

10. The title *Waṣīya* features in a quotation by Ibn al-Muṭrān (see Ullmann, *Medizin im Islam,* 162); for Abū al-ᶜAlāʾ's literary activity, see ibid., 162–63; and Álvarez Millán, "Actualización del corpus médico-literario de los Banū Zuhr," 173–80.

11. For Abū Marwān b. Zuhr (d. 1162) and Maimonides' high regard for him, see Maimonides, *On Asthma* 9.1; Ullmann, *Medizin im Islam,* 162–63; and Álvarez Millán, "Actualización del corpus médico-literario de los Banū Zuhr," 173–80.

12. See aphorisms 13.44–49, 51.

and, similarly, to drink it with wine. Those who compound this remedy [and administer it] are mistaken, because they want to strengthen the organs and let the medicine rise to the head; but [they] forget that the effect of these purgatives is carried to the major organs, and sometimes such an organ cannot tolerate this, and [the patient] is killed" (aphorism 13.49), Maimonides comments:

> This is correct if the purgation is done by poisonous drugs, such as pulp of colocynth or turbith [*Ipomoea turpethum*], because of their poisonous effect; or [by strong drugs, such as] laurel [*Laurus nobilis*], because of its strength. But safe drugs—and especially agaric, which is good for poisons—are very beneficial if imbibed in wine. I have done so several times [and used such a drug] in order to cleanse the head, and [I] saw that it is very effective and that it cleanses the brain to a degree any [other] drug is incapable of. Moreover, the patient taking this drug found [new] energy and dilation of the soul. Therefore, consider the specific properties of the drugs that you administer. (aphorism 13.50)

Sometimes Maimonides quotes from inauthentic Galenic treatises, as is the case for his quotations from Pseudo-Galen's commentary on Hippocrates' *De humoribus*.[13] These quotations are a valuable source for reconstructing part of Galen's genuine commentary to this book since the text edited by Kühn is, as Deichgräber showed, a Renaissance forgery.[14] On that occasion Deichgräber also demonstrated that Maimonides' quotations closely parallel those of Oribasius, but at the same time he warned against too much optimism, since both Maimonides and Oribasius tend to abbreviate the original Galenic text.[15] Another Pseudo-Galenic quotation is found in aphorism 14.9: "If it is easy for someone to vomit, he should do so before [taking] food, in order to cleanse his body from the superfluities of the [previous] food [he took]. If it is difficult for someone to vomit, he should vomit after [taking] food, in order to cleanse his body from the phlegm as well. *In Hippocratis De mulierum affectibus commentarius.*"

Galen's commentary on Hippocrates' *Diseases of Women* is of doubtful authenticity since it is mentioned by only Ibn Abī Uṣaybiʿa, not by Ḥunayn ibn Isḥāq.[16] However, Maimonides' quotation is certainly inauthentic

---

13. See aphorisms 12.43; 13.20, 29, 37; 14.3.

14. Deichgräber, *Hippokrates' "De humoribus,"* 43; cf. the translator's introduction to the second volume of Maimonides, *Medical Aphorisms,* ed. and trans. Bos.

15. Deichgräber, *Hippokrates' "De humoribus,"* 45.

16. Ibn Abī Uṣaybiʿa, *ʿUyūn al-anbāʾ fī ṭabaqāt al-aṭibbāʾ,* 149. Cf. Meyerhof, "Schriften Galens," 542, no. 56; Ullmann, "Zwei spätantike Kommentare," 245–62;

because its subject bears no relation to women's diseases; such a collection of unrelated and thus inauthentic prescriptions already features in the Hippocratic text itself.[17]

As I showed in the introduction to the edition of *Medical Aphorisms: Treatises 1–5*, in many cases Maimonides not just reproduces the Galenic text, but rather reformulates it through abbreviation or addition. A telling example of an abbreviation is found in the chart below, comparing aphorism 10.36, where Maimonides quotes from Galen's *De inequali intemperie* 8,[18] with Ḥunayn's Arabic translation of Galen:[19]

Maimonides, *Medical Aphorisms* 10.36	Galen, *Fī sū' al-mizāj al-mukhtalif*, MS Ayasofya 3593, fol. 52a
الحّمى التي تعرض فيها إحساس الحرّ والبرد معا ويوجد الحرّ الشديد مع النافض البارد سبب ذلك إذا كثر في البدن البلغم الزجاجي والخلط الذي من جنس الصفراء حتّى يغلبان معا على البدن ويتحرّكان في الأعضاء الحسّاسة	وذلك أنه ليس شيء من هذا بجب. ولا كيف تعرض الحّمى والنافض لبعض الناس في حال واحدة من قبل أنه إذا كثر في البدن الخلط البارد البلغي الذي يشبهه فكسا غورس بالزجاج والخلط الحارّ الذي من جنس الصفراء حتّى يغلبا معا على البدن ويتحرّكا فيه وخاصّة في الأعضاء الحسّاسة فليس بجب أن يحسّ من تلك حاله بالأمرين جميعا. فإنّك إن عمدت إلى إنسان فآقمته في شمس حارّة ثمّ رششت عليه ماء باردا فليس من المحال أن يحسّ بحرارة الشمس وبرد الماء إلّا أنّ هذين جميعا إنّما تاله من خارج وناله أيضا كلّ واحد منهما في أجزاء من بدنه عظيمة.

and the translator's introduction to the first volume of Maimonides, *Medical Aphorisms,* ed. and trans. Bos.

17. See Littré, ed., *Oeuvres complètes d'Hippocrate,* 1:92–109.

18. See ed. Kühn, 7:749–50.

19. Forthcoming edition of the Arabic text and the Hebrew and Latin translations, edited by Gerrit Bos, Michael McVaugh, and Joseph Shatzmiller.

| **Maimonides,** *Medical Aphorisms* **10.36** | **Galen, *Fī sū' al-mizāj al-mukhtalif*, MS Ayasofya 3593, fol. 52a** |

٢. وأمّا الحمّى التي يسمّيها اليونانيون
انفيالس فالذي يناله من الحرّ والبرد إنّما
يناله من داخل ويناله أيضًا كلّ واحد
منهما في أجزاء بدنه الصغار حتّى يكون
الأوّل ليس من بدنه أجزاء عظيمة ينالها
البرد إلّا إلى جانب كلّ واحد منها جزء
عظيم يناله الحرّ ويكون الثاني ليس من بدنه
جزء صغير يناله البرد إلّا وإلى جانبه جزء
آخر صغير يناله الحرّ ولذلك صار هذا
الثاني يظنّ أنّه يحسّ في بدنه كلّه بالأمرين
جميعًا وذلك لمّا كان كلّ واحد من المبرد
والمسخن مبثوثًا في أجزاء صغار

حتّى لا يبقى من بدنه جزء صغير يناله البرد
إلّا ولجانبه جزء صغير آخر يناله الحرّ،
فيحسّ من داخل بدنه بالحرّ والبرد معًا لأنّ
كلّ واحد من المسخن والمبرد مبثوثًا في أجزاء
صغار جدًّا. في مقالته في سوء المزاج

The reason that, in some fevers, a sensation of heat and cold occurs simultaneously, and that one finds high fever and cold rigor, is that the vitreous phlegm and the yellow bile increase so much that together they dominate the body and move through the sensitive parts of the body

Nor [is it amazing] how fever and rigor occur to some men at the same time, for if the cold phlegmatic humor that Praxagoras compares to glass and the hot humor that belongs to the same kind as yellow bile increase in the body until together they dominate and move in it, especially in the sensitive organs, it is not amazing that someone who has this disposition senses both at once. For if you approach a man and let him stand in the hot sun, and then sprinkle cold water over him, it is not impossible that he should feel the heat of the sun and the cold of the water [together]. But these two affect [that man] in that situation only from the outside, and each of them affects him [only] in the large parts of his body.

| Maimonides, | Galen, *Fī sū' al-mizāj al-mukhtalif*, |
| Medical Aphorisms 10.36 | MS Ayasofya 3593, fol. 52a |

2. But in the fever which the Greeks call "enpialos" [epialos], heat and cold affect [the patient] from the inside, and each one of them may affect [the patient] [not only in the large parts] but also in the small parts of his body. This happens to a degree that in the first case (i.e., the patient affected in the large parts), there is no large part of his body affected by cold, unless next to it there is [another] large part affected by heat; and in the second case (i.e., the patient affected in the small parts), there is no small part affected by cold, unless next to it there is another small part affected by heat. Therefore it happens, in the second case, that [the patient] seems to sense both things together in his body. And this is because, as everything that cools and heats is scattered through small parts . . .

until every small part affected by the cold has, next to it, another small part affected by the heat. Someone suffering from this feels heat and cold inside his body at the same time because both the heating and the cooling [humors] are dispersed throughout the smallest parts [of the body]. *De [inequali] intemperie.*

An example of an addition is aphorism 10.50, where Galen remarks: "When a patient craves inhaling cold air because he has the sensation of a severe burning in the inner parts of his body, yet needs many clothes [to warm his body] from the outside because of the cold he feels, it is a sign that his illness is fatal," and Maimonides comments: "unless it occurs in the beginning of the [fever] attacks."[20] And in aphorism 12.35, Galen advises bloodletting from the left arm for an illness of the spleen, and Maimonides adds that the vein to be bled is the basilic one. On another occasion Maimonides evaluates a general rule by Galen for bloodletting in the case of melancholic delusion as "a most important diagnostic rule" (aphorism 12.40). And, as we saw above in the case of Abū al-ʿAlāʾ ibn Zuhr, Maimonides' additions sometimes assume the form of an explicit comment, introduced by "Says Moses" (*qāla Mūsā*).

---

20. Of course, one cannot discard the possibility that such a reading was part of the Galenic text Maimonides consulted.

All these additions are of primary importance for our evaluation of Maimonides' theoretical and practical medical knowledge, especially in the field of pharmacology, a subject in which Maimonides was particularly interested.[21] Thus, in aphorisms 13.2–3, when Galen remarks that "compound purgatives are bad when one of the ingredients has a purgative effect as soon as the purgative enters the body, while another ingredient has this effect only long after its ingestion," Maimonides adds that "latex plants and scammony purge as soon as they arrive in the body, whereas purgative resins purge only after a [prolonged] period." Maimonides also remarks that these resins are opopanax, galbanum, sagapenum, asafetida, and gum ammoniacum. And in aphorism 13.6, after repeating Galen's recommendation to rinse the stomach after taking a purgative with barley gruel or groats, Maimonides comments that "the consumption of barley groats, once the effect [of the purgatives] has worn off, is something unusual in all the countries I have passed through," and that "it causes nausea, because the stomach quickly needs to throw up [even] after the [effect of the] purgative [has worn off]."

As we have already seen, Maimonides did not turn a blind eye to inconsistencies or contradictions in the works of Galen, his much-revered master.[22] In aphorisms 15.3–4, Maimonides quotes Galen's statements that cauterization should only be applied to those bodily parts that do not have depth—i.e., hands, feet and loins—and that, in the case of lung ulcers, the chest should be cauterized when one cannot cleanse the lungs through expectoration. He then remarks in 15.5 that these two statements would have been mutually exclusive if Galen had not explicitly stipulated under which exceptional circumstances cauterization to the chest is allowed. However, when on another occasion Galen recommends a quick cauterization to the chest in the case of dropsy patients suffering from lung ulcers, without any further stipulation that might classify this case as exceptional (a text quoted by Maimonides without any further comment in aphorism 15.7), Maimonides attacks him for being inconsequential: "In his commentary to *De aere and aquis* 2 he says: 'One should not cauterize a part of the body except the hands, feet and loins.' But in book 7 of his commentary on *Epidemics* 6, he says: 'Those who suffer from lung ulcers should be quickly cauterized on their chests.' These are his

---

21. See the translator's introduction to Maimonides, *On Asthma* (ed. and trans. Bos) and Bos, "Maimonides' Medical Works and their Contribution," 246–48.

22. See the translator's introduction to the first volume of Maimonides, *Medical Aphorisms*, ed. and trans. Bos.

very words and they annul his previous statement. Consider this" (aphorism 25.18).

Finally, the importance of a critical edition of Maimonides' *Medical Aphorisms* based on all the available manuscripts can be demonstrated by examining Deller's translations of Maimonides' quotations from Galen's *Commentaries on Hippocrates' Epidemics*. His translation is sometimes faulty because it is based on a corrupt version found in the only manuscript consulted for the Arabic text: MS Leiden 128.1. An example of such a corruption is provided in aphorism 10.37:

> There are two kinds of rigor that do not abate until the time of the climax draws near. One of them is that which does not abate until the climax of the *fever attack* is near. This one is malignant, but not severe, and originates from the putrefaction of the very cold phlegm called "vitreous." The other one is that which does not abate until the climax of the *entire illness* is near, for quartan fever cannot reach its climax until the rigor lessens. The rigor that begins with great severity and then abates before the time of the climax is that which happens in the case of tertian fever. *In Hippocratis Epidemiarum* 6.1.

Instead of "The other one is that which does not abate" (*la yaskun*), he translates *"Die zweite Art wird erhitzt"* (The second kind is heated), following the corruption of MS Leiden: *yaskhun*. And in aphorism 10.45, where Galen speaks about ardent fever accompanied by a diarrhea of raw material (*ikhtilāf nīʾ*), Deller, following manuscript L's version, *ikhtilāf qaiʾ*, translates *"verbrennendes Fieber mit Erbrechen"* (ardent fever accompanied by vomiting).[23]

Manuscripts of the
Kitāb al-fuṣūl fī al-ṭibb (Medical Aphorisms)

The work is known to be extant in the following manuscripts:

1. Gotha 1937 (**G**); fols. 6–273 (fol. 7 numbered twice); Naskh script.[24] A considerable section of the text, from treatise 6.10 (beginning at *al-mawt*) to treatise 7.16 (ending at *min amthāl*), is missing.[25] Other sections, namely 20.30–33 and 23.7, 13, 15, 69, and 82, seem to have been missing

---

23. See as well the translator's introduction to Maimonides, *Medical Aphorisms: 6–9*, ed. and trans. Bos.

24. See Pertsch, *Orientalischen Handschriften*, 3:477–78; Kahle, "Aphorismorum praefatio et excerpta," 89–90.

25. Other sections missing are 20.30–33 and 25.56–58.

from the original version used by the scribe and were added by him at the end of these treatises from another version. According to the colophon on fol. 273a, which appears after aphorism 25.55, the scribe copied the text from a copy of the original redaction of the work by Maimonides' nephew Abū al-Maʾālī (or Maʾānī) ibn Yūsuf ibn ʿAbdallāh.[26] The scribe adds that he found a note in the text at hand in which Abū al-Maʾālī remarks that, in the case of the first twenty-four *maqālat*, Maimonides would correct his autograph notes and that he, Abū al-Maʾālī, would then make a fair copy and correct it in Maimonides' presence; however, the text of the twenty-fifth *maqāla* was copied by him in the beginning of the year 602 AH (August 1205 AD), after the death of Maimonides, so the latter had not been able to do the redaction.[27] Although it is generally agreed that this manuscript has preserved the best readings,[28] it should be noted that in some cases the text suffers from a certain carelessness by the scribe, resulting in mistakes and corruptions. Moreover, the language he employs is sometimes extremely vulgar and colloquial. Another characteristic of the text is that the central issue of many aphorisms is indicated in the margin, using terminology derived from the text itself.

2. Leiden 1344, Or. 128.1 (**L**); 140 fols.; Maghribī script.[29] The manuscript ends on fol. 140b with the following colophon:

> This is the end of the treatise—praise be to God—and the completion of the Book of Aphorisms of the most perfect and unique scholar Mūsā ibn Maymūn ibn ʿUbaydallāh, the Israelite, from Cordova—may God be pleased with him. The copying [of the text] was completed in the month of May of the year 1362, according to the calendar of al-Ṣufr, in the city of Ṭulayṭula—may God protect it—and it was written by Yūsuf ibn Isḥāq ibn Shabbathay, the Israelite.

---

26. See the remark by the scribe at the end of **G**, treatise 24 (fol. 239a): "Something like the following was written at the end of this treatise: This is what I found in the copy written by Abū [...]: I did not make a fair copy of this treatise until after his death—may God have mercy on him—and [A]bū al-Zakāt the physician wrote: Praise be to God, who is exalted."

27. See Pertsch, *Orientalischen Handschriften,* 3:477–78; Kahle, "Aphorismorum praefatio et excerpta," 90; Kaufmann, "Neveu de Maimonide," 152–53; Meyerhof, "Medical Work," 276; Kraemer, "Six Unpublished Maimonides Letters," 2:79–80 n. 93; Sirat, "Liste de manuscrits du Dalālat al-ḥayryn," 4:112; Stern, ed. and trans., *Maimonides' Treatise to a Prince,* 18.

28. Cf. Schacht and Meyerhof, "Maimonides against Galen," 59; Maimonides, *Medical Aphorisms,* trans. Rosner, xiv.

29. See Voorhoeve, *Handlist of Arabic Manuscripts,* 85.

The calendar of al-Ṣufr was common in Spain, especially among Christians, and started about thirty-eight years before the Christian calendar.[30] Accordingly, the manuscript was written in May 1324 in Toledo. More than any of the other manuscripts, the language of this manuscript conforms to the rules of classical Arabic; the influence of vulgarization is thus far less pronounced than in the others. Just like **G**, it has many marginal catchwords.

3. Paris, Bibliothèque nationale, héb. 1210 (**P**); 130 fols.; Judeo-Arabic; no date.[31] The manuscript only contains treatises 1–9 (the last one incomplete), part of treatise 24, and the major part of treatise 25. Also missing is 8.42–59. According to the inscription on fol. 1v, the manuscript was once in the possession of R. Meir ha-QNZ(?)Y. The text has been copied carefully, so that there are only a few mistakes; the top section has been so stained that the first lines are hard to read.

4. Escorial, Real Biblioteca de El Escorial 868 (**E**); fols. 117–26 (numbered in reverse order); Maghribī script.[32] According to the colophon this text was copied in the city of Qalᶜa (Alcalá) by Mūsā ibn Sūshān al-Yahudī in the year 1380 (read 1388), corresponding to the year 5149 since the creation. The text offers a close parallel to **L**, both having many otherwise unique readings in common, including whole paragraphs not appearing in any other manuscript, as, for instance, aphorism 3.52. Like **L**, it has several marginal catchwords, but they are not as many and they use a different terminology.

5. Escorial, Real Biblioteca de El Escorial 869 (**S**); fols. 176–1 (numbered in reverse order); Oriental script; no date.[33] The text finishes at aphorism 25.58 and is missing an important section between 10.28 (from المستدل) and 21.73. The text of this manuscript is closely related to **G**.

6. Oxford, Bodleian, Uri 412, Poc. 319, cat. Neubauer 2113 (**B**); 123 fols.; Judeo-Arabic; Sephardic semicursive script.[34] According to the

---

30. See Dozy, *Supplément aux Dictionnaires arabes,* 1:836; Kahle, "Aphorismorum praefatio et excerpta," 90–91.

31. See Zotenberg, ed., *Catalogues des Manuscrits hébreux et samaritains,* 223; Vajda, *Index général des manuscrits arabes musulmans,* 345.

32. See Derenbourg, comp., and Renaud, ed., *Les manuscrits arabes de l'Escorial,* vol. 2, fasc. 2, pp. 74–75; Cano Ledesma, *Indización de los manuscritos árabes,* 65, no. 33; Koningsveld, "Andalusian-Arabic Manuscripts," 102 n. 87.

33. See Derenbourg, comp., and Renaud, ed., *Les manuscrits arabes de l'Escorial,* vol. 2, fasc. 2, p. 76; Cano Ledesma, *Indización de los manuscritos árabes,* 65, no. 33.

34. See Neubauer, *Hebrew Manuscripts in the Bodleian Library,* 721; see as well Beit-Arié and May, *Supplement of Addenda and Corrigenda,* col. 392.

colophon, the text was copied by Makhluf ben Rabbu Shmuʾel he-Ḥazan DMNSY (from Mans?) and completed on the eleventh of Elul 5112 (1352 AD).[35] Numerous Hebrew versions derived from Nathan ha-Meʾati's Hebrew translation have been added to the text above the lines and in the margins. The text suffers from many omissions and corruptions but does provide some unique variant readings—as, for instance, in treatise 3.22: المرك—a unique, correct version according to Galen's τῆς συνθέτου σαρκὸς.[36]

7. Oxford, Bodleian, Hunt. Donat 33, Uri 423, cat. Neubauer 2114 (**O**); 78 fols.; Sephardic semicursive script; ca. 1300(?)[37] The text begins with treatise 23, continues with 6.90 (from إذا طالات) to treatise 24 (incomplete, large sections missing), and ends with 12.

The colophon found at the end of book 12 reads:

كتب المقالة التاسعة عشر وعدد فصولها ألف الحد لله على حسن ع <...> والسلام على
المألفين من الله <...> تمّ الكّاب في سنت الف ט"ג لחרבן ב"ש תם

The flyleaf at the beginning reads:

הדה אלכתאב יסמא כתאב אלפצול לאן אנמזג' קול אטבא והו שרח אלמוג'ז והו כתאב יסמא
אלדכיראת אלאטבא בג'מעאהן לגאלינוס ופצולהו ואבא קראט ופצ'להו צחא וקול אלחכים מוסא
אלקורטבי ופצול אבן זהר ועדד ופצולהון אללף פצל פי אלטב ואמראץ' אלרדן מן אלראס ללקדם פי
עלם אלאבדאן מנלראס לחד אלאקדאם ופצול באלאכואץ לעלאג' אל נאס.

The flyleaf at the end by the same hand reads:

כתאב אלדי כאן ענתי פי מצר נאקלתו פי סאלופכי' פי זמאן צלטן עצמן תריך ע'ה'ע'ס' סנת אלדי
כונת פי אליגורנא מע דודור מורין ורחונא לאליגורנא קדנא שהירין ורחות אנא ומעלמי לאנגלאאתירא
קדנא סני וג'ינא עלא ויניזיא .קדנא שהר וג'ינא לשיו פי סנת ה' ותלאתמיי" ותלאתין וכמס'. תאריך.

The text has a few catchwords, some in Judeo-Arabic and some in Arabic. The beginning and end have been falsified and the original figures of the chapters have been altered. This manuscript is closely related to **E** and **L**, sharing many characteristic readings.

---

35. Beit-Arié and May, *Supplement of Addenda and Corrigenda,* col. 392, states that Steinschneider refers to "a physician by the name of Makhluf of Marsala, Syracuse (Sicily)."

36. Galen, *De usu partium* 12.3 (ed. Helmreich, 2:188 line 4).

37. See Neubauer, *Hebrew Manuscripts in the Bodleian Library,* 722; Beit-Arié and May, *Supplement of Addenda and Corrigenda,* col. 392.

8. Oxford, Bodleian, Hunt. 356, Uri 426, cat. Neubauer 2115 (**U**); 107 fols., Oriental semicursive script; late thirteenth century.[38] The manuscript itself provides us with two dates on fol. 106b: 1535, and a second date that is hard to decipher—possibly the year 1500. The text runs from treatise 10.5 (at الضرورة) until 24.27 and has the following colophon:

תמת אלמקאלה י"ה בעון מאלך אלדוניה אלחכים עלא אל ספלייה ואלעלאויה וחאכים עלא עלאוייה
ואל ספלייה צחיב אל דוניה אל מצ'ייא. שנת ה'ר'צ'ה.

The text on the flyleaf at the beginning reads:

האדא לשמעון אלחכים אלמערוף באבן חנין אלראיס פי מדינת בגדאד אלמערוף בל עלם פל טב
כתאב כט אבי עזרא רחמהו אלה קד נקלו מן כתאב קדים.

A second text on the same flyleaf reads:

האדא אלכתאב אלעזיז אלשריף לחביש אלתפפליסי ומפראתו פל אדויה מתעלקה באכואץ אלצחיחה
ואלמעדין ועדד אלפצול סתמאיה וסתה וסבעון בעון אלחי אלחק אלקיום קד אן כתאב פי מדינה
באביל פי שנת ה'ק'ג'ה'. כתבתו(?) באיבירייא ובאירחמן ארחם[...].[39]

The text on the flyleaf at the end (fol. 107a) reads:

תמאת מקאלה חביש אלתפפליסי אלמערוף אבן חבש אלחכים אלעריף אלזאהיר אלמאהיר אלעריף
באלתקים ואלתלטיף אלכביר אלחר'ף עדד מקאלתהו סתה מאיה וסתה וסבעין פל אדויה ואלמפרדאת
[...] אלמקאלת ועדד אלפצול מגמוע גמיע סימן תהעו בעון [...] רחמאן.[40]

Just as in the previous manuscript, the beginning and end have been falsified. Similarly, the headings and figures of the chapters have been altered.[41]

9. Göttingen 99. This manuscript was copied by Antonius Deussingius in the year 1635 in Leiden from **L**.[42]

10. Istanbul Velieddin 2525.[43]

---

38. See Neubauer, *Hebrew Manuscripts in the Bodleian Library,* 722; Beit-Arié and May, *Supplement of Addenda and Corrigenda,* col. 392.

39. [...] כתבתו(?) באיבירייא ובאירחמן ארחם: Missing in Neubauer, *Hebrew Manuscripts in the Bodleian Library,* 722; Beit-Arié and May, *Supplement of Addenda and Corrigenda,* col. 392.

40. Missing in Neubauer, *Hebrew Manuscripts in the Bodleian Library,* 722; Beit-Arié and May, *Supplement of Addenda and Corrigenda,* col. 392.

41. See Langermann, *Synochous Fever,* 185 n. 24.

42. See Kahle, "Aphorismum praefatio et excerpta," 89.

43. See Ullmann, *Medizin im Islam,* 167 n. 4. I was unable to obtain photocopies of this manuscript.

For the edition of Maimonides' *Medical Aphorisms: Treatises 10–15*, the following manuscripts have been consulted: Gotha 1937 (**G**), Leiden 1344 (**L**), Escorial 868 (**E**) and 869 (**S**; until 10.28), and Oxford 2113 (**B**), 2114 (**O**), and 2115 (**U**). These manuscripts can be divided into two main groups, namely, **SG** and **EBLOU**. The edition is mainly based on MS Gotha 1937.

The decision to edit *Medical Aphorisms* in Arabic characters, rather than in Hebrew ones, has been inspired by Maimonides' own practice. Recent scholarship gives reason to assume that Maimonides usually composed a first draft of his medical works, intended for private use, in Arabic written in Hebrew characters, and that these works were subsequently transcribed into Arabic characters when intended for public use. Thus Stern remarks that "all of Maimonides' medical works were naturally published in Arabic script, since otherwise they would have been of no use to the non-Jewish public," and adds that Maimonides first drafted the text in Hebrew script, because the Hebrew script was easier for him, and then had it transcribed into the Arabic script.[44] Stern's point of view has been endorsed by Hopkins, who remarks that although we have sporadic autograph examples of his Arabic handwriting, Maimonides always used the Hebrew script when writing privately.[45] Other scholars have expressed somewhat different opinions in this matter. Meyerhof remarks that Maimonides composed all of his medical writings in Arabic, probably using Arabic characters, since he had nothing to hide from the Muslims.[46] Blau suggests that when addressing a general public, including Muslims and Christians (as in the case of medical writings), Jewish authors might have used Arabic script; but when addressing a Jewish audience, they wrote in Hebrew characters.[47] Langermann remarks that it seems likely that many of Maimonides' medical writings were originally written in Arabic characters and that only afterwards were these transcribed into Hebrew characters.[48]

For editing the Arabic text, which is written in Middle Arabic typical for this genre, I have adhered to the guidelines formulated by Oliver

---

44. See Stern, ed. and trans., *Maimonides' Treatise to a Prince*, 18; cf. comments by Blau, *Emergence and Linguistic Background of Judaeo-Arabic*, 41 n. 6.

45. See Hopkins, "Languages of Maimonides," 90.

46. Meyerhof, "Medical Work," 272.

47. Blau, *Emergence and Linguistic Background of Judaeo-Arabic*, 41; cf. Baron, *Social and Religious History of the Jews*, 8:403 n. 42.

48. Langermann, "Arabic Writings in Hebrew Manuscripts," 139.

Kahl. Morphological and syntactical and even grievous offences against the grammar of classical Arabic have been neither included in the apparatus nor changed or corrected at all. Orthographical peculiarities have not been included in the critical apparatus either. They have been either adjusted to the conventional spelling or left in their original forms, as the need for clarity dictated.[49]

As with *Medical Aphorisms: Treatises 1–5* and *Medical Aphorisms: Treatises 6–9*, this edition is supplemented by a list of faulty readings and translations selected from Muntner's edition[50] of Nathan ha-Meʾati's Hebrew translation[51] and from Rosner's English translation.[52] Muntner's edition is based on a corrupt manuscript: Paris, Bibliothèque nationale, hébr. 1173,[53] and therefore has many errors. Since Rosner's translation follows Muntner's edition, it suffers from many mistakes as well. The list also provides the versions of these particular readings by Zeraḥyah ben Isaac ben Sheʾaltiel Ḥen (**Z**), derived from his translation of the *Medical Aphorisms*.[54] I also noted a few examples of faulty readings by Zeraḥyah and correct ones by Nathan. It is my hope that on the basis of this list and ideally on the basis of future critical editions of these translations, it will be possible to provide critical evaluations of the translation activity of these two prominent medieval translators. With this goal in mind, a supplemental volume containing a comparative Arabic-Hebrew-English glossary of technical terms used in *Medical Aphorisms* is being planned. The Hebrew terms will also be listed alphabetically in separate indexes with reference to the comparative glossary. Thus, the glossary and indexes may contribute to our our knowledge of the medieval Hebrew

---

49. See Kahl's edition of Sābūr ibn Sahl, *Dispensatorium parvum,* 35–38.

50. Maimonides, *Pirḳei Mosheh bi-refuʾah,* ed. Muntner.

51. Nathan ha-Meʾati (from Cento) prepared this translation in Rome between 1279 and 1283. For his data see Vogelstein and Rieger, *Geschichte der Juden in Rom,* 1:398–400; Steinschneider, *Hebräischen Übersetzungen des Mittelalters,* 766; Freudenthal, "Sciences dans les communautés juives," 69.

52. Maimonides, *Medical Aphorisms,* ed. Rosner.

53. See Zotenberg, *Catalogues des manuscrits hébreux et samaritains,* 215.

54. For Zeraḥyah's versions I consulted MS Munich 111. On Zeraḥyah, who was active as a translator in Rome and who prepared the translation of the *Medical Aphorisms* in 1279, see Vogelstein and Rieger, *Geschichte der Juden in Rom,* 1:271–75, 409–18; Ravitzky, "Mishnato shel R. Zeraḥyah," 69–75; ch. 7, "Zeraḥyah's Technique of Translation," in Bos, ed., *Aristotle's "De Anima" Translated into Hebrew;* Freudenthal, "Sciences dans les communautés juives," 67–69; Zonta, "Hebrew Translation of Hippocrates' De superfoetatione," 104–9.

medical terminology. They may also be used to amplify dictionaries of the Hebrew language or, ideally, to create a dictionary devoted to this particular area. During the compilation of the glossary, it became increasingly clear that both of the Hebrew translations are based on an Arabic text represented by manuscripts **E** and **L**, since they share several unique readings. As explained in the first volume of *Medical Aphorisms,* Zerahyah's translation is characterized by many terms in Latin and Romance, and these will be registered in a separate index.

Last but not least, at the end of this volume I have also provided a list of addenda and corrigenda to the first two volumes, resulting from the preparation of an edition of the Hebrew translation by Zerahyah. The publishers have also included some corrections to the sigla found in the introduction to volume 2.

MEDICAL APHORISMS

TREATISES 10–15

◆

In the name of God,
the Merciful, the Compassionate.
O Lord, make [our task] easy

The Tenth Treatise

Containing aphorisms concerning fevers

(1) When the digestion of the foods in the stomach and liver is not as thorough as it should be, fevers increase and become sharper. Therefore, in the case of all fevers, one should pay the utmost attention to the [proper] digestion of the food through strengthening the stomach and liver with astringent things.[1] *De methodo [medendi]* 11.[2]

(2) Do not permit those suffering from fever to drink enough water to quench their thirst until you have thoroughly looked into the matter. When one of the noble organs is afflicted by an inflamed tumor [alone], or an inflamed tumor combined with erysipelas, or a soft or hard tumor; or when the body of the patient has an obstruction or a putrefaction of uncocted humors; or when it has an organ with a cold temperament, which is always harmed by cold water—in all these cases, the patient should not be given cold water to drink until there are clear signs that the putrefying humors are being cocted or that the inflamed tumor has

بِسْمِ اللهِ الرَّحْمَنِ الرَّحِيمِ

رَبِّ يَسِّرْ

المقالة العاشرة

تشتمل على فصول تتعلق بالحميات

١. الأغذية متى لم يستحكم انهضامها كما ينبغي في المعدة والكبد تزيدت الحميات ٥
واشتدّت حدّتها. ولذلك ينبغي أن يعنى أشدّ عناية في جميع الحميات باستمراء الغذاء
بتقوية المعدة والكبد بالأشياء القابضة. حادية عشر الحيلة.

٢. لا تقدم على إباحة المحمومين شرب الماء البارد قدر ريهم حتى تستقصي
النظر. فمتى كان في أحد الأعضاء الشريفة ورم فلغموني أو فلغموني مخالط للحمرة
أو ورم رخو أو صلب أو كان بالمريض سدد أو كان في بدنه عفونة من أخلاط لم ١٠
تنضج أو كان في بدنه عضو بارد المزاج يتضرّر دائما بالماء البارد فكل واحد من
هؤلاء لا ينبغي أن يسقى ماء باردا حتى تتبيّن علامات نضج الأخلاط العفنة أو نضج

_____

١ بسم الله الرحمن الرحيم ربّ يسّر] om. ELBO || ٦ أن يعنى] om. B || ٨ قدر
ريهم] om. B || ٩ الأعضاء] G¹ | مخالط للحمرة] حمرة E || ١٠ سدد] سدة B ||
١١ البارد] om. ELO

— ١ —

become ripe. Someone suffering from a true erysipelas should be treated through the ingestion of cold water [under the same conditions].[3] *De methodo [medendi]* 9.[4]

(3) In the case of putrid fevers, you should consider and look into three things: the strength [of the patient], which is the most important;[5] then the cause of the putrefaction; and, finally, the fever itself. If you find that the agents with which you want to treat the fever are good for [all] these three things, it is very good.[6] But if you find that one or more than one agent has a contrary effect on one or more than one of these three things, set your mind on that which maintains and supports the strength. Sometimes you should treat only the cause—namely, when the heat of the fever is weak—and attempt to open the obstruction and to combat the putrefaction. But when the fever is flaring up somewhat, attempt to extinguish the heat of the fever, even if you increase the obstruction. For, sometimes, the fever is so exceptionally high that a human being quickly perishes therefrom because he cannot bear or endure it. *De methodo [medendi]* 10.[7]

(4) If we knew the [different] natures of fevers[8] for certain, we could risk telling many fever sufferers to bathe in cold water [at home] and not only in the bathhouse, and some might benefit from that. But since we do not have a real and exhaustive knowledge of the [different] natures of fevers, and since a mistake therein at an inopportune occasion could lead to great harm, we avoid this therapy in the treatment [of fever patients]. *De methodo [medendi]* 10.[9]

If a young man who is well-fleshed and corpulent and does not suffer from an inflammation[10] in his viscera takes a bath in cold water and swims therein during the time of the summer heat and the culmination of the fever, he [clearly] benefits from [such treatment], and I recommend this without hesitation. *De methodo [medendi]* 10.[11]

الورم الفلغموني. وأمّا من كان معه ورم حمرة خالص فداوه بشرب الماء البارد. تاسعة الحيلة.

٣. ينبغي أن تجعل بحثك وقصدك في الحمّيات العفنية ثلاثة أشياء القوة وهي أوّلها وآخرها وبعدها سبب العفونة ثمّ نفس الحمّى. فإن وجدت الأشياء التي تداوي بها موافقة لثلاثتها فذاك وإن خالفت بعضها بعض فتوخّ ما يبقى القوة ويرفدها. وقد تداوي السبب وحده إذا كانت حرارة الحمّى ضعيفة فتعني بتفتيح السدد ومقاومة العفونة. وإن شبّت الحمّى قليلا وقد تعني بطئ حرارة الحمّى وإن زدنا في السدّة لأنّه ربّما كانت الحمّى في الندرة بها من العظم ما يتلف به الإنسان سريعا ولا يقدر على احتمالها والصبر عليها. عاشرة الحيلة.

٤. لوكّا من معرفة طبائع الحمّيات على يقين لكّا سنجسر أن نأمر كثيرا من المحمومين بالاستحمام بالماء البارد من غير حمّام وقد استفع بذلك قوم. لكّا لمّا كّا لا نعرف طبائع الحمّيات بالحقيقة والاستقصاء وكان الغلط في ذلك إن وقع في غير موضعه يعقب ضررا عظيما صرنا نتجنّب هذه الأشياء في المداواة. عاشرة الحيلة.

لوأنّ رجلا شابّا حسن اللحم خصب البدن في وقت القيظ في وقت منتهى من حمّى وليس في أحشائه ورم استحمّ بماء بارد وسبح فيه لانتفع بذلك ونحن نأمر بهذا بلا توقّف. عاشرة الحيلة.

١ الورم] الدم B | فداوه بشرب] فدواه شرب LO || ٣ العفنية] العفونية EL : العفنة
B | القوة وهي أوّلها وآخرها] وهي أوّلها وأوكدها القوة L : القوة وهي أوّلها وأكدها
S || ٤ وبعدها] وبعده EL || ٥ فذاك] فذلك ESL : S² : فذاك S² | فتوخّ] فتودا B : فتوّف
L || ٧ وإن] زاد SG¹ add. : B add. كان | شبّت] سبب SGB || ١٠ الحمّات] الحمّى
ESGLO || ١٣ نتجنّب] نجتنب ELBO || ١٤ من حمّى] من الحمّى L : الحمّى EB

(5) If you find it necessary to bleed a fever patient,[12] or to purge him, or to alleviate the pain he is suffering from with a poultice or a hot compress, you should not give him barley groats or barley gruel before doing the aforementioned. *In Hippocratis De acutorum morborum [victu] commen-*
5   *tarius* 1.[13]

(6) The factor[s] that determine the length or brevity of a fever attack, even if there is only one kind of fever [present], is the condition of that humor that putrefies and bursts forth by itself, and the condition of the expulsive faculty, and the condition of the passages and channels of
10   the organ close to that humor. A surplus or thickness or viscosity of that humor necessarily makes the attack lengthy, while the opposite makes the attack short. Similarly, a weak expulsive faculty makes the attack lengthy, and a strong expulsive faculty makes it short; and narrow passages and channels make it lengthy, and wide passages and channels
15   make it short. Sometimes all the factors determining the lengthiness [of the attack] coincide, and sometimes all the factors determining the shortness [of the attack] coincide. *De [differentiis] febrium* 2.[14]

(7) A fever arising from the putrefaction of humors has its own specific symptom that always goes with it—namely, a quick contraction of
20   the [pulsatile] vessels [of the wrist].[15] This becomes especially evident during the increase of the fever attack, although it is not imperceptible during its beginning and climax. At its beginning, the pulse is small; and at its climax, it is great. *De [differentiis] febrium* 1.[16]

(8) If someone whose body is full [of humors] is attacked by fever
25   and then by diarrhea, [no other kind of evacuation is needed].[17] This is sufficient for him, even if it is not commensurate with the degree[18] of fullness of his body. If someone attempts to bleed such a person or make his diarrhea more severe, he brings him into immediate danger. *Ad Glauconem [de methodo medendi]* 1.[19]

30   (9) If someone who has only recently suffered from indigestion is attacked by fever when he has a feeling of biting and pressure in the cardia of his stomach and while his body is full of blood, one should not attempt to bleed him before paying attention to the cardia of his stomach. When

٥. المحموم إن دعتك الضرورة أن تقصده أو تسهله أو تسكّن وجعا به بضماد أو تكميد وليس ينبغي أن تنيّله كشك الشعير ولا ماؤه دون أن تفعل به ذلك. في شرحه لأولى الأمراض الحادّة.

٦. السبب في طول نوبة الحمّى وقصرها وإن كان نوع تلك الحمّى واحدا هو حال ذلك الخلط الذي يتعفّن ويندفع في نفسه، وحال القوة الدافعة وحال مجاري العضو الحاوي لذلك الخلط ومنافذه. وذلك أنّ كثرة الخلط أو غلظه أو لزوجته توجب طول النوبة وأضداد ذلك توجب قصرها. وكذلك ضعف القوة الدافعة يوجب طول النوبة وشدّة القوة توجب قصر النوبة وضيق المجاري والمنافذ يوجب طول النوبة وسعتها توجب قصر النوبة. وقد تجتمع أسباب الطول كلّها وقد تجتمع أسباب القصر كلّها. في الثانية من الحمّيات.

٧. الحمّى المتولّدة عن عفونة الأخلاط لها دليل خاصّ بها لا يفارقها وهو سرعة انقباض العرق، وذلك يظهر ظهورا بيّنا في وقت تزيّد نوبة الحمّى وليس هو بالخفي في وقت الابتداء ووقت الانتهاء. وفي وقت ابتدائها يكون النبض صغيرا وفي وقت المنتهى يكون عظيما. في الأولى من الحمّيات.

٨. من عرضت له حمّى وهو ممتلئ وحدث به ذرب فيكتفى به وإن لم يكن بحسب مقدار امتلاء بدنه. ومن قدم على إخراج الدم لهم أو يزيد في إسهالهم فيكسبهم خطرا عاجلا. أولى أغلوقن.

٩. من أصابته حمّى وكان قريب العهد بالتخمة ويجد لذعا وعصرا في فم معدته وكان في بدنه امتلاء من الدم فلا تقدم على فصده حتّى تقدم العيانة بفم معدته،

---

it[s condition] has improved, one may evacuate the whole body. I have often seen how physicians evacuated [the bodies of] patients with this condition without first strengthening the stomach. Some of [the patients] died, and others became so dangerously ill that they were on the verge of death. *Ad Glauconem [de methodo medendi]* 1.[20]

(10) If putrefaction occurs in the viscera or large vessels, something similar to the vapor of the humors that have putrefied there reaches the two chambers of the heart. However, in the case of swollen glands[21] or of tumors in any soft, fleshy part [of the body], only the heat spreads from there to the heart and warms the surrounding region. The heat continues to spread until it reaches the heart and heats it, without any vapor of the putrid humor reaching the heart together with it, because that humor is confined [to those places]. Therefore, the first [case] concerns putrid fever; and the second, ephemeral fever. *De [differentiis] febrium* 1.[22]

(11) Cold in the extremities, especially during fevers, [occurs] either because of a large, inflamed tumor in the viscera; or because of a severe pain in the middle part of the body;[23] or because of fainting or syncope;[24] or because of weakness of the innate heat and its near extinction; or because of its drowning and choking effect[25] due to a surplus of [superfluous] matters. The extremities are the ears, nose, hands, and feet. *In Hippocratis Aphorismos commentarius* 7.[26]

(12) When cold occurs in the extremities in the beginning of fever attacks, it is not a fatal sign. However, it indicates that blood and heat [first] gather inside the body and then spread. *In Hippocratis Prognostica commentarius* 2.[27]

(13) When cold and pallor of the extremities occur in combination with acute fever, it indicates death and extinction of the innate heat. *In Hippocratis Epidemiarum librum* 3 *commentarius* 2.[28]

(14) When cold sweat occurs together with acute fever, it is a sign of death. *De signis mortis.*[29]

(15) Sometimes putrefaction occurs in all the vessels equally, but sometimes it occurs [only] in the largest and most eminent vessels— namely, those between the groins and the armpits. This putrefaction is necessarily the root of continous fever. When putrefaction occurs [only]

فإذا انصلحت استفرغت البدن كلّه. وقد رأيت مراراً كثيرة من هذه حاله قد استفرغهم الأطباء قبل تقوية المعدة. بعضهم هلك وبعضهم بلغ به الخطرأن أشرف على الهلاك. أولى أغلوقن.

١٠. متى كانت العفونة في الأحشاء أو في العروق الكبار فإنه يتأدى إلى بطني القلب شي شبيه بالدخان من الأخلاط التي تتعفّن هناك. وأمّا أورام الحالبين أو ورم أيّ لحم رخو فإن الحرارة فقط تسري منه إلى القلب بكونه يسخن ما يليه. ولا تزال الحرارة حتّى تصل إلى القلب فتسخنه من غير أن يصل معها إلى القلب شيء من بخار ذلك الخلط العفن لكون ذلك الخلط محصورا. ولذلك كانت الأولى حتى عفنية وهذه الثانية حتى يوم. أولى الحمّيات.

١١. بردالأطراف خاصّة في الحمّيات إمّا من قبل ورم عظيم في الأحشاء أو من قبل وجع شديد في الجوف أو من ذبول النفس والغشي أو من قبل خمول الحرارة الغريزية وقرب انطفائها أو من قبل انغمارها أو اختناقها بكثرة المواد. والأطراف هي الأذنان والأنف والكفّان والقدمان. في شرحه لسابعة الفصول.

١٢. ليس برد الأطراف في ابتداء نوائب الحمّى دليل هلاك وإنما هو دليل على انقباض الدم والحرارة إلى داخل ثمّ تنتشر. في شرحه لثانية تقدمة المعرفة.

١٣. برد الأطراف وخضرتها إذا كان مع حمّى حادّة فهو يدلّ على موت الحرارة الغريزية وانطفائها. في ثانية شرحه لثالثة أبيديميا.

١٤. العرق البارد مع الحمّى الحادّة دليل على الموت. في مقالته في علامات الموت.

١٥. العفونة قد تكون في عروق كلّها بالسوى وقد تكون في أعظمها وأشرفها وهي العروق التي فيما بين الحالبين والإبطين وهذه ضرورة تكون أصل الحمّى المطبقة.

---

in one organ with an [inflamed] tumor—or even without one—the root and source of the fever are in that organ. This putrefaction is to the fever as a blazing fire.[30] *De methodo [medendi]* 11.[31]

(16) One should know which remedies are good for curing a fever,
5   which are good for treating putrefaction, and which are good for treating the cause of putrefaction—namely, an obstruction. The remedies good for the treatment of these three [things] are not always compatible. On the contrary, it often occurs that the effect of one of these remedies is contrary to that of the other[s]. One should look for the most severe and
10   harmful of these three [things] and treat it first. *De methodo [medendi]* 11.[32]

(17) You should know for certain that differentiation[33] between fever, putrefaction, and its cause (when [also] present) is abstruse, difficult, and hard. [Discerning] it requires a subtle mind and a refined intellect. It is even harder to differentiate between these and the strength [of the body].
15   *De methodo [medendi]* 11.[34]

(18) If someone suffers from fever while his body contains a very large quantity of crude superfluities and his stomach has been weakened through indigestions, his body appears swollen. The complexion of some of [these patients] becomes white or dark or lead-colored, and their pulse
20   becomes small and unequal. These patients should not be phlebotomized under any circumstances, nor can they tolerate purgation of the bowels, even if they need evacuation. If one of these methods is applied to them, they are overcome by syncope. They only benefit from an evacuation by means of strong massage, which brings the patient to near-exhaustion
25   because of the bruising of the flesh through the intensive massage. One should stop massaging these patients during sleep, because sleep cocts [the superfluities], whereas wakefulness causes [their] dissolution. If someone falls ill because of crude humors, he should be treated equally with these two methods. *De methodo [medendi]* 12.[35]

30   (19) There are three kinds of intermittent fevers that stop in a perceptible way: tertian fever, quotidian fever, and quartan fever. Tertian fever originates from yellow bile when it putrefies; quotidian fever originates from humors that strongly tend to become like phlegm when they putrefy; and quartan fever originates from melancholic humors when

أمّا إذا كانت العفونة في عضو واحد به ورم وليس فيه ورم فإنّ أصل تلك الحمّى ومعدنها في ذلك العضو وهي للحمّى بمنزلة نار المستوقد. حادية عشر الحيلة.

١٦. ينبغي أن تعلم أيّ الأشياء هي التي تداوى بها الحمّى وأيّ الأشياء هي دواء للعفونة وأيّها دواء لسبب العفونة أعني السدد. فإنّ الأشياء التي تداوى بها هذه الثلاثة ليست بمتّفقة دائما بل كثيرا ما يضادّ بعضها بعضا. فتقصد أعظم هذه الثلاثة وأشدّها نكاية وتفضّله في المداواة. حادية عشر الحيلة.

١٧. ينبغي أن تعلم علما يقينا أنّ المقايسة بين الحمّى والعفونة والسبب الفاعل للعفونة، إن كان حاضرا، أمر خفيّ شاقّ عسر ويحتاج إلى ذهن لطيف وعقل مهذّب. وأشدّ من ذلك مشقّة أن يقايس بين هذه وبين القوّة. حادية عشر الحيلة.

١٨. من أصابته الحمّى وفي بدنه فضل خام كثير جدّا ومعدته قد أضعفتها التخم فإنّ هذا يرى بدنه ينتفخ. وبعضهم يصير لونه أبيض أو أسود أو رصاصي وبعضهم صغيرا مختلفا. وهؤلاء لا تقصد لهم عرقا بوجه ولا يحتملون أيضا إسهال البطن وإن كانوا محتاجين إلى الاستفراغ. ومتى فعل بهم أحد هذين تخلّلهم الغشي. ولا يصلح لهم غير الاستفراغ بالدلك الشديد الذي يكاد أن يحدث الإعياء لترضيض اللحم بكثرة الدلك، واقطع دلكهم عند النوم لأنّ النوم ينضج واليقظة تحلّل. ومن كان مرضه من أخلاط نيئة فهو محتاج إلى هذين باعتدال. ثانية عشر الحيلة.

١٩. أصناف الحمّيات المفارقة التي تقلع إقلاعا محسوسا ثلاثة وهي الغبّ والنائبة في كلّ يوم والربع. والغبّ تتولّد من المرّة الصفراء إذا عفنت، والنائبة في كلّ يوم تتولّد من أخلاط هي إلى البلغم أميل إذا هي عفنت، والربع تتولّد من أخلاط سوداوية إذا

---

٢ المستوقد] مستوقد ELO ‖ ٤ دواء] التي تداوى بها EO ‖ ١٨ في كلّ يوم] EO ‖ ١٩ من] عن EO ‖ om. S

they putrefy. When the humor that produces the fever streams throughout the body, these three kinds [of fevers] are clearly intermittent. *De [differentiis] febrium* 2.[36]

(20) Continuous fevers occur when the putrid humor that produces the fever is confined within the vessels—this humor is one of the three humors.[37] The continuous fever that does not end on the third day but rather becomes worse is similar to tertian fever and is the [so-called] continuous tertian fever. And the type that does not end nor depart but occurs every day in the same way is the [so-called] continuous quotidian fever. This fever does not have a clear end. The same applies to continuous quartan fever, which becomes worse on the fourth day, but which [only] rarely occurs. *De [differentiis] febrium* 2.[38]

(21) Even when a continuous fever is difficult to move[39] and stretches up to forty days, it is still counted among the acute diseases. And even when it really passes away [and recurs], it is also counted among the chronic diseases. When I said "a continuous fever," understand that I mean a fever that does not really pass away. *De diebus decretoriis* 2.[40]

(22) One of the most important symptoms for putrid fever is the quality of its heat: it always bites and smarts, just like the effect of smoke on the eyes. Nothing at all is pleasant about it, not even in the beginning of its attacks, when the heat has not yet spread. If you leave your hand for a long time on the body, the heat ascends and, even more, bites and hurts. In its beginning, one never finds cocted urine; rather, [it is] uncocted or cocted in a very obscure way.[41] One does not find compression of the pulse or of the heat in nonputrid fevers. Nevertheless, [their occurrence] is not specific for putrid fevers alone. *De differentiis febrium* 1.[42]

(23) Sometimes [the quality of] the blood changes when it putrefies: it turns into yellow bile or black bile. In these cases, the fever is either tertian or quartan. The only difference between these cases is that in the first one,[43] the fever is malignant; but when it originates from the transformation of the blood, it is not malignant. For when the heat tends more toward the vaporous type and is less aggressive and harmful

هي عفنت. وإذا كان الخلط المولّد للحمّى جاريا في البدن كلّه كانت هذه الثلاثة أنواع مفارقة بيّنة الإقلاع. ثانية الحمّيات.

٢٠. الحمّيات الدائمة هي التي يكون الخلط العفن المولّد للحمّى محصورا داخل العروق، وهي من هذه الأخلاط الثلاثة. فما كان منها لا يقلع ويشتدّ في الثالث فهي الشبيهة بالغبّ وهي الغبّ الدائمة. وما كانت لا تقلع ولا تفارق ولكنّها تنوب كلّ يوم على مثال واحد فهي النائبة في كلّ يوم الدائمة ولا يتبيّن لها إقلاع. وكذلك يكون ربع دائمة وهي تشتدّ في الرابع، وهذه قليل ما تقع. ثانية الحمّيات.

٢١. الحمّى الدائمة وإن كانت حركتها ثقيلة وتمتدّ إلى الأربعين فهي أيضا تعدّ من الأمراض الحادّة. وإن كانت الحمّى تقلع فيها إقلاعا صحيحا فهي أيضا تعدّ من الأمراض المزمنة. وإذا قلت حمّى دائمة فافهم عنّي أنّها لا تقلع إقلاعا صحيحا. ثانية أيّام البحران.

٢٢. من أعظم دلائل حمّيات العفونة كيفية الحرارة فيها لأنّها أبدا تلذع وتقرض مثل فعل الدخان للعينين، وليس فيها لذاذة أصلا ولو في ابتداء نوائبها الذي لم تنشر الحرارة حينئذ. وإذا طال لبث كمّك على البدن ارتفعت الحرارة الغير لذيذة بل تقرض وتؤلّم. ولا يوجد فيها أبدا في الأوّل بول نضيج بل عادم النضج أو أثره خفيّ جدّا ولا يوجد تضاغط النبد أو تضاغط الحرارة في غير العفنة وليس هذا خاصّ بها وحدها. في أولى الحمّيات.

٢٣. وقد ينقلب الدم إذا عفن فيصير صفراويا أو سوداويا فتكون الحمّى من نوع الغبّ أو من نوع الربع وليس بينهما فرق إلّا أنّ تلك خبيثة وهذه الكائنة عن انقلاب الدم ليست بخبيثة. فإنّ الحرارة متى كانت أميل إلى البخارية وأقلّ عادية وأذى

---

٦ في] om. ELBOU | الدائمة] دائما B || ٨ إلى ألأربعين] للأربعين ELU : لأربعين O || ١٣ للعينين] G¹

when one touches [the body], it comes from [the transformation of] the blood; but when it is biting and smarting when one touches [the body], it comes from the putrefaction of [one of] the two biles. And if one touches the body and does not find sharpness in the beginning, but [later], when one leaves one's hand on it for a long time, one has a sensation of biting that slowly increases and is uneven, so that it feels as if it were transmitted through the holes of a filter or a sieve, then heat originates from the putrefaction of the phlegm. This humor cannot be dissolved from the body evenly because of its thickness and viscosity. *De [differentiis] febrium* 2.[44]

(24) The cycle of phlegmatic fever[45] is twenty-four hours; the cycle of tertian fever is forty-eight hours; and that of quartan fever, seventy-two hours. This is clear. For, [in the case] of phlegmatic fever, which attacks every day, there are twenty-four hours from the beginning of the first attack until the beginning of the second attack. The same analogy can be made for tertian and quartan fevers. If, for instance, you find an eight-hour cycle in which the attacks last for six hours and then remit for two hours and then return in the same manner and remit again for two hours, continuously, you know that this is a case of a threefold phlegmatic fever, because the eight hours represent one-third of the cycle of the phlegmatic fever. Similarly, if you find a cycle every sixteen hours, you know that this is a case of a threefold tertian fever, because the sixteen hours are one-third of the cycle of tertian fever. If you find a cycle of eighteen hours, you know that it is a fourfold quartan fever, because eighteen hours are one-fourth of the cycle of quartan fever. *De circuitibus febrium.*[46]

(25) The pulse does not return to its natural state in any of the other fevers, not even if a very long interval [occurs] between the first and the second attack, such as the interval that occurs between the attacks in the cases of tertian and quartan fevers. For, in the cases of those fevers, the symptoms of the fever remain in the vessels, except for quotidian fever. [In the case of this fever], the symptoms of the fever disappear and vanish when the fever subsides. *Ad Glauconem [de medendi methodo]* 1.[47]

للمس فهي من الدم. ومتى كانت لذّاعة قارضة للمس فهي عن عفن المرتين. ومتى كان
أوّل ما تلمس البدن لا تجد حدّة فإذا طال لبث كفّك عليه أحسست بتلذيع يتزيد
قليلا بعد قليل وفيه اختلاف حتّى كأنّها تنفذ من أثقاب مصفاة أو منخل فتلك الحرارة
عن عفن البلغم لأنّ هذا الخلط لغلظه ولزوجته لا يتحلّل المتحلّل من بدنه على السوى.

٥ ثانية الحمّيات.

٢٤. دور الحمّى البلغمية أربعة وعشرون ساعة ودور الغبّ ثمانية وأربعين ساعة
ودور الربع اثنين وسبعين ساعة وهذا بيّن. وذلك أنّ الحمّى البلغمية التي تنوب كلّ يوم
من أوّل النوبة الأولى إلى أوّل النوبة الثانية أربعة وعشرون ساعة. وكذلك هو
القياس في الغبّ والربع. فإن وجدت مثلا دورا ثماني ساعات مثل أن تدوم النوبة
١٠ ستّة ساعات وتفارق ساعتين ثمّ تنوب كذلك وتفارق ساعتين على الاستمرار فتعلم
أنّ هذا معه ثلاث حمّيات بلغمية لأنّ الثمان ساعات هي ثلث دور الحمّى البلغمية.
وكذلك إن وجدت دورا كلّ ستّ عشر ساعة فتعلم أنّ به ثلث حمّيات غبّ لأنّ
الستّ عشر ساعة ثلث دور الغبّ. فإن وجدت دورا ثمان عشر ساعة علمت أنّ
به أربع حمّيات ربع لأنّ ثمان عشر ساعة ربع دور الربع. في مقالته في أدوار الحمّيات.

١٥ ٢٥. ليس يعود النبض في شيء من سائر الحمّيات الى حاله الطبيعية ولا إن كان
بين ابتداء النوبة الأولى والثانية زمان طويل جدّا كالزمان الذي بين ابتداء نوائب
حمّيات الغبّ والربع. وذلك أنّ في تلك الحمّيات لا يزال دليل الحمّى باقيا في العروق إلا
حمّى يوم، فإنّ دليل الحمّى يبطل ويمتنع مع سكون الحمّى. في الأولى من أغلوقن.

___

٦ دور] G¹ || ١٤ ساعة] S² : om. G

(26) The regularity in the cycles of a fever is disrupted and altered for one of two reasons: either because of an alteration from one nature to another of the humors that produce the fever, or because of an error in the diet. Sometimes one may think that a fever does not have a certain regularity, while [in reality] it does. [This happens because the fever] is composed of many cycles, but the physician does not notice its composite character. *De [differentiis] febrium* 2.⁴⁸

(27) Sometimes [the intervals between] every fever attack occurring from the beginning until the end of a disease are the same, whether the attack comes early or late after the preceding one. The physicians call those early ones "early cycles" and the opposite ones "late cycles." The earliness or lateness thereof does not indicate a strengthening of the disease nor its decline. Rather, it should be taken as an indication of the shortness or length of the attack and of the malignity or badness of the symptoms or the disappearance of these symptoms. *De crisibus* 1.⁴⁹

(28) The indications for pure tertian fever (which can be derived from the observation of the patient himself in the beginning of the attack) are eleven:

1. A severe rigor whereby one has the sensation of needle pricks.

2. Thirst and burning heat that do not last long.

3. An equal pulse, whatever its condition.

4. A quick climax to the attack.

5. Equal distribution of the heat through the entire body.

6. Abundant and sharp heat at the first contact of the hand with the body, then a decline as the heat is overcome by [the heat of] the hand.

7. The passage of a hot vapor through the pores [of the body] during the drinking of water.

8. The emesis of bile or the excretion of bile through diarrhea or through urine in which the bile dominates (sometimes all three occur at the same time).

٢٦. يفسد نظام أدوار الحمّى ويختلف لأحد سببين: إمّا من قبل انقلاب الأخلاط المولّدة للحمّى من طبيعة إلى طبيعة وإمّا من قبل خطأ يعرض في التدبير. وقد يظنّ بالحمّى أنها غير لازمة لنظام وهي لازمة لنظام. وسبب ذلك كونها أدوارا كثيرة مركّبة لم يشعر الطبيب بتركيبها. في ثانية الحمّيات.

٢٧. قد تكون الحمّى من أوّل المرض إلى آخره كلّ نوبة تتقدّم على التي قبلها على نسبة ٥ واحدة أو تتأخّر، ويسمّون الأطبّاء تلك المتقدّمة أدوارا متقدّمة ويسمّون خلافها أدوارا متأخّرة. ولا يدلّ تقدّمها ولا تأخّرها لا على تزيّد المرض ولا على انحطاطه. وإنّما يعتبر ذلك بقصر مدّة النوبة وطولها وبخباثة الأعراض ورداءتها أو بارتفاع تلك الأعراض. أولى البحران.

٢٨. علامات حمّى الغبّ الخالصة المستدلّ بها من نفس مباشرة المريض أوّل ١٠ نوبة أحد عشر علامة:

(١) النافض القوي الذي يحسّ فيه بنخس الإبر.

(٢) العطش والتلهّب ولا يطول ذلك.

(٣) استواء النبض على أيّ حال كان.

(٤) انتهاء النوبة في أسرع زمان. ١٥

(٥) انتشار الحرارة في البدن كلّه بالسوى.

(٦) كثرة الحرارة وحدّتها أوّل لقاء الكفّ للبدن ثمّ تفور الحرارة ويقهرها الكفّ.

(٧) نفوذ بخار حارّ من المسامّ عند شرب الماء.

(٨) قيء المرار أو اختلاف مرار أو بول يغلب فيه المرار، وقد تجتمع ثلاثتها. ٢٠

---

١٠. الخالصة] MS S ends here ‖ ١٢ القوي] السو ELO ‖ نخس] بغرز ELOU ‖
١٨ ويقهرها] ويرقّها B

9. Even perspiration over the whole body.

10. Alleviation and complete disappearance of the fever.

11. The longest period for the total fever attack being twelve hours, and the shortest, six hours. *De crisibus* 2.[50]

(29) The indications for pure quartan fever that can be derived perfectly well from the fever itself are four:

1. All the indications for pure tertian fever are absent; moreover, most of the indications that one finds for quartan fever are the opposite of those for pure tertian fever.

2. Quartan fever rarely begins first; rather, it [mostly] occurs after other fevers.

3. The pulse of such patients is transformed in the beginning of the attack and becomes like the pulse of a very old man, unlike the pulse of patients suffering from any other kind of fever.

4. It begins simply, with a mild rigor that becomes stronger with every attack. With every rigor, the patient feels a cold whose severity matches the severity of the rigor, until he feels, when it is severe, as if his bones were being crushed by snow. *De crisibus* 2.[51]

(30) The indications for quotidian fever that are clear, evident, and easy to obtain are seven:

1. It does not begin with a rigor on the first day, and as time passes, the patient has, in the beginning of the attack, a sensation of cold in the outer part of his body and the extremities, but not a real rigor.

2. Inequality and irregularity of the pulse [occur] mostly in the beginning of the attack.

3. [There is no] burning heat; the heat and thirst are so little that the thirst is less than in the other fevers.

4. Its patients hardly perspire during the first days, while their urine is uncocted.

5. It mostly occurs with pain of the cardia of the stomach and of the liver.

(٩) العرق المستوي في البدن كلّه.

(١٠) سكون الحمّى وإقلاعها إقلاعا تامّا.

(١١) أطول مدّة النوبة كلّها إثنى عشر ساعة وأقصرها ستّ. ثانية البحران.

٢٩. علامات الربع الخالصة المستدلّ بها من نفس الحمّى على التحميل أربع علامات:

(١) عدم علامات الغبّ الخالصة كلّها بل أكثرها يوجد في الربع على خلاف ما هي في الغبّ الخالصة.

(٢) أنّ الربع قلّ ما تبتدئ أوّلا وإنّما تكون بعد تقدّم حمّيات آخَر.

(٣) إنّ نبض أصحابها في أوّل النوبة ينقلب ويصير كنبض الشيخ الهرم ولا يوجد نبض أحد من المحمومين كذلك.

(٤) إنّما تبتدئ بنافض ضعيف ثمّ تقوى في كلّ نوبة. وكلّ نافض يحسّ فيه بيرد شديد على قدر شدّة النافض حتّى يحسّ منه عند اشتدادها كأنّ العظام ترضّ بالثلج. ثانية البحران.

٣٠. علامات الحمّى النائبة في كلّ يوم البيّنة الظاهرة السهلة الإدراك سبعة:

(١) إنّها لا تبتدئ من أوّل يوم بنافض وكلّما تمادَت الأيّام يحسّ في أوّل النوبة بيرد ظاهر البدن والأطراف لا بنافض حقيقي.

(٢) إختلاف النبض وعدم الانتظام وأكثر ذلك في أوّل النوبة.

(٣) عدم التلهّب وقلّة الحرارة والعطش حتّى أنّ العطش فيها أقلّ منه في سائر الحمّيات.

(٤) كونها لا يكاد يعرق فيها في الأيّام الأوّل مع فجاجة البول حينئذ.

(٥) كون أكثر حدوثها مع ألم فم المعدة والكبد.

---

٣ ستّ] ساعات ‖ ٦ ساعات] add. EL ‖ ٧ آخر] om. ELBOU ‖ ٨ ينقلب] ينقل L

6. The hypochondria swell and increase in the beginning of the occurrence of the fever.

7. The face[s] of its sufferers [are] yellowish-white, even at the time of the climax of the attack. *De crisibus* 2.[52]

(31) In every continuous fever, the [putrefying] matter is inside the [nonpulsatile] vessels. It is not accompanied by rigor, or perspiration, or emesis. A fever originating from a bloody tumor is a mild and safe one and very similar to ephemeral fever, which originates from a tumor in the soft flesh in the groin and other places. *De crisibus* 2.[53]

(32) When various causes of fever occur simultaneously, begin [treatment] with bleeding through phlebotomy, and then start to dilute and thin the humors, and then [work] to soften the solid matter and to rarefy contracted spots of the skin.[54] *De methodo medendi* 11.[55]

(33) [Galen] said on the general treatment of tertian fever: "If signs of coction appear, confidently administer some absinthe to the patient because it has a laudable effect in different respects. Moreover, it is one of the most adequate means for the treatment of diseases developing at the cardia of the stomach from the biting [effect] of bile." *Ad Glauconem [de medendi methodo]* 1.[56]

(34) At its inception, tertian fever begins with severe rigor. As for quartan fever, I do not know that I [ever] saw[57] that it started with severe rigor. But, in the case of this fever, the rigor becomes more severe as time passes and mostly originates from what remained from other preceding fevers and from the fever called "the mixed one."[58] *Ad Glauconem [de medendi methodo]* 1.[59]

(35) When pure tertian fever lasts as long as possible, it ends after seven cycles. In spite of this, it is one of the least dangerous fevers. But when it is impure, the situation is the reverse. I know that this fever once started in a young man in the beginning of autumn and did not leave him until spring. *Ad Glauconem [de medendi methodo]* 1.[60]

(٦) انتفاخ ما دون الشراسيف وعظمه أوّل حدوث الحمّى.

(٧) كون وجه المريض بين البياض والصفرة ولو عند منتهى النوبة.

٣١. كلّ حمّى دائمة تكون مادّتها داخل العروق ولا يكون معها نافض ولا عرق ولا قيء. والحمّى التي تتولّد عن الورم الدموي حمّى لينة سليمة وهي أشبه شيء بحمّى يوم العارضة عن ورم اللحم الرخو الذي في الحالب وغيره من المواضع. ثانية البحران.

٣٢. إذا اجتمعت في وقت واحد أسباب شتّى من أسباب الحمّى فتبتدئ بإخراج الدم بالفصد، ثمّ تأخذ في تلطيف الأخلاط وترقيقها، ثمّ في تليين ما تكبّز وتخفيف ما انقبض من الجلد. حادية عشر الحيلة.

٣٣. قال في جملة علاج حمّى الغبّ فإن ظهرت علامات النضج فثق وتقدم على إعطايته شيء من الأفسنتين فإنّه له عملا محمودا من وجوه، وهو مع ذلك من أبلغ ما يتعالج به في العلل التي تحدث في فم المعدة من تلذيع المرار. أولى أغلوقن.

٣٤. الغبّ أوّل حدوثها تبتدئ بنافض شديد وأمّا الربع فلا أعلم أنّي رأيتها ابتدأت بنافض شديد. وإنّما يشتد النافض فيها ويصعب على طول الأيّام، وفي أكثر الأمر إنّما يحدث عن بقية من حميات آخر تقدمها وعن الحمّى التي تسمّى المختلطة. في أولى أغلوقن.

٣٥. حمّى الغبّ الخالصة انقضاؤها يكون على أطول ما يكون في سبعة أدوار وهي مع ذلك من أسلم الحميات من الخطر. ومتى كانت غير خالصة ولا نقية فالحال فيها على خلاف ذلك. وإنّي لا أعلم أنّ هذه الحمّى ابتدأت مرّة بغلام في أوّل الخريف فلم تقارقه إلى الربيع. في أولى أغلوقن.

---

٢ منتهى] المنتهى G || ٧ تكبّز] تلين L : تقبّض O || ٩ فثق] om.O : فقد L || ١٢ أنّي] متى ELBOU || ١٤ تقدمها] تقدّمتها ELBU : تتقدّمها O || ١٦ على] om. L || أطول] أفضل B

(36) The reason that, in some fevers, a sensation of heat and cold occurs simultaneously, and that one finds high fever and cold rigor, is that the vitreous phlegm and the yellow bile humor increase so much that together they dominate the body and move through the sensitive parts of the body until every small part affected by the cold has, next to it, another small part affected by the heat. Someone suffering from this feels heat and cold inside his body at the same time because both the heating and the cooling [humors] are dispersed throughout the smallest parts [of the body]. *De [inequali] intemperie.*[61]

(37) There are two kinds of rigor that do not abate until the time of the climax draws near. One of them is that which does not abate until the climax of the *fever attack* is near. This one is malignant,[62] but not severe, and originates from the putrefaction of the very cold phlegm called "vitreous." The other one is that which does not abate until the climax of the *entire illness* is near, for quartan fever cannot reach its climax until the rigor lessens. The rigor that begins with great severity and then abates before the time of the climax is that which happens in the case of tertian fever. *In Hippocratis Epidemiarum* 6.1.[63]

(38) In pure tertian fever, the longest duration of an attack is twelve hours. In an impure tertian fever, it can last for twenty or twenty-four hours. In some cases this fever has an extremely long attack, lasting about forty hours, whereas its abatement lasts for eight hours. All this goes back to what we mentioned above, about the causes of the length of an attack. *De [differentiis] febrium* 2.[64]

٣٦. الحمّى التي تعرض فيها إحساس الحرّ والبرد معا ويوجد الحرّ الشديد مع النافض البارد سبب ذلك إذا أكثر في البدن البلغم الزجاجي والخلط الذي من جنس الصفراء حتّى يغلبان معا على البدن ويتحرّكان في الأعضاء الحسّاسة حتّى لا يبقى من بدنه جزء صغير يناله البرد إلا ولجانبه جزء صغير آخر يناله الحرّ، فيحسّ من داخل

٥ بدنه بالحرّ والبرد معا لأنّ كلّ واحد من المسخّن والمبرّد مبثوثا في أجزاء صغار جدًا. في مقالته في سوء المزاج.

٣٧. النافض الذي لا يسكن حتّى يقرب المنتهى ضربان: أحدهما الذي لا يسكن حتّى يقرب منتهى نوبة الحمّى وهو خبيث وليس بشديد وهو يعرض عن عفن البلغم القوي البرودة الذي يسمّى الزجاجي. والضرب الآخر هو الذي لا يسكن حتّى يقرب

١٠ منتهى المرض كلّه فإنّ حمّى الربع لا يعلم أنّها قد بلغت منتهاها حتّى يبتدئ النافض يتناقص. والنافض الذي يبتدئ بشدّة شديدة ثمّ يسكن قبل وقت المنتهى يكون في حمّى الغبّ. في الأولى من شرح سادسة أبيديميا.

٣٨. الغبّ الخالصة أكثر ما تكون نوبتها إثني عشر ساعة، وأمّا الغبّ الغير خالصة فقد تطول نوبتها عشرين ساعة وأربعة وعشرين ساعة. وقد تكون غبّ زائدة الطول جدًا تطول نوبتها نحو أربعين ساعة والراحة ثمانية ساعات. كلّ هذا راجع

١٥ لما تقدّم ذكره من أسباب طول النوبة. في ثانية الحمّيات.

---

١ ويوجد] وبجد ELOU: وتجد O || ٣ يبقى] G¹ || ٨ يقرب] يقدم L || ٩ لا يسكن] لا يسخن ELO || ١٢ أبيديميا] أفيديميا ELO

(39) If a patient suffers from two tertian fevers and two quintan fevers, the two tertian fevers attack daily, and the two quintan fevers attack on the third day. Therefore, one might think that the two tertian fevers are a single quotidian fever and that the two quintan fevers are a single tertian fever. *De crisibus* 2.[65]

(40) Ardent fevers hardly ever originate from the congestion of yellow bile, but, rather, from the domination of the heat[66] in the vessels when it [the yellow bile] becomes sharp and inflamed through the condition of the air,[67] physical exercise, hot dishes, or movements of the soul. *In Hippocratis Epidemiarum* 1.2.[68]

(41) One should first examine the nature of the fever—whether its heat is strong, blazing, and ardent. A fever with such a condition has its crisis with evacuation. When a fever is mild and weak, similar to a smoldering fire,[69] it can last for a long time, and its crisis mostly occurs with abscesses. *Ad Glauconem [de medendi methodo]* 1.[70]

(42) The worst ardent fevers are those which occur because of the liver or stomach. They can also occur because of [inflamed] tumors in the lung or because of bilious humors that putrefy and spread through the entire body and that, because of their putrefaction, become exceedingly hot, similar to a boiling process. *De locis affectis* 5.[71]

(43) One of the worst indications is when an acute, ardent fever occurs or when a hot, sharp superfluity streams to the stomach but does not incite thirst. For this indicates that the sensatory faculty in the stomach has stopped functioning and has died. *In Hippocratis Epidemiarum* 1.1.[72]

٣٩. إن كان بالمريض حميان غبّ وحميان خمس فإنّ الغبّين نائبان في كلّ يوم
والخمسان نائبان غبّا. فيظنّ بالغبّين أنهما حمّى واحدة في كلّ يوم ويظنّ بالخمسين
أنهما غبّ واحدة . ثانية البحران.

٤٠. الحمّيات المحرقة لا يكاد تتولّد من احتقان المرّة الصفراء، وإنّما تكون من غلبة
الحرارة التي تكون في الأوعية إذا احتدّت والتهبت عن حال الهواء أو رياضة
أو أطعمة حارّة أو حركات نفسانية. في ثانية شرح الأولى من أبيديميا.

٤١. ينبغي لك أن تنظر أوّلا في طبيعة الحمّى هل هي قوية الحرارة ملتهبة محرقة
فما حاله هكذا من الحمّيات فبحرانها باستفراغ. وما كان من الحمّيات ليّنا رقيقا شبيها
بالنار المدفونة فمن شأنها أن تطول وبحرانها على الأمر الأكثر بالخراجات. في
الأولى أغلوقن.

٤٢. الحمّيات المحرقة أشدّها ما كان بسبب الكبد والمعدة وقد تكون أيضا بسبب
أورام الرئة أو بسبب أخلاط مرارية تعفن وتنتشر في جميع البدن وتصير بسبب
عفونتها إلى الحرارة المفرطة الشبيهة بالغليان. خامسة التعرّف.

٤٣. من أعظم العلامات خبثا أن تكون حمّى حادّة محرقة أو تكون يتجلّب إلى
المعدة فضل حارّ حادّ فلا يحدث عطشا لأنّ هذا يدلّ أنّ القوة الحسّاسة التي في
المعدة قد بطلت وماتت. في الأولى من شرحه للأولى من أبيديميا.

---

١ نائبان] يأتيان U || ٢ نائبان] يأتيان U || ٥ تكون] om.ELBOU | حال الهواء] هواء
ELOU || ٦ أبيديميا] أفيديميا ELOU || ٧ ينبغي...أبيديميا (٤٦)] om. E || ١٢ أو]
إذا هي ورمت ورما من جنس الورم المعروف بالحمر كما أنها قد تكون L | تنتشر في جميع
البدن] om. L || ١٤ حادّة] = ¹L : واحدة L || ١٦ أبيديميا] أفيديميا LO : أبديميا B

(44) When the humor that causes the fever is sharp and burning, a tumor hardly ever develops in the area of the ears. When the humor is extremely cold and thick, tumors develop in the lower parts of the body. When the humor is in the middle, between these two conditions, tumors
5   develop beneath the ears. *In Hippocratis Epidemiarum* 2.2.[73]

(45) Sometimes ardent fever is accompanied by a diarrhea of raw material. This is caused by the presence of raw humors in the vessels connected to the intestines and in the concave side of the liver. When ardent fever is accompanied by thin urine, it indicates the presence of
10   many uncocted humors in the the convex side of the liver. *In Hippocratis Epidemiarum* 3.2.[74]

(46) There are two accurate indications for ardent fever: constant thirst, which does not stop or abate, and a blazing heat so intense that it can be felt through touching.[75] *In Hippocratis Epidemiarum* 3.3.[76]
15   (47) When all the three faculties [of the body] are strong while there is a severe ardent fever and there are clear, evident signs of coction, give the patient cold water to drink with trust and confidence, unless he is a very old man. *De methodo [medendi]* 12.[77]

(48) Ardent fever develops from the putrefaction of yellow bile in
20   the stomach and especially in its cardia, or in the concave side of the liver, but not in any [other] organ. One of the most specific properties of ardent fever is that its crisis comes through a nosebleed, because the blood ascends and rises,[78] whereat the [nonpulsatile] vessels burst open. *In Hippocratis Epidemiarum* 1.1.[79]
25   (49) Ardent fevers develop from either yellow bile or salt phlegm. *In Hippocratis De acutorum morborum [victu] et Galeni commentarius* 3.[80]

٤٤. إذا كان الخلط المولّد للحمّى حادّا محترقا فلا يكاد يحدث ورم عند الآذان. وإذا كان الخلط شديد البرودة والغلظ حدثت الأورام في أسافل البدن. وإذا كان الخلط متوسّطا بين الحالين حدثت الأورام تحت الآذان. في الثانية من شرحه لثانية أبيديميا.

٤٥. قد يكون مع الحمّى المحرقة اختلاف نيء. وعلّة ذلك أنّه يكون في العروق التي تتّصل بالأمعاء وفي الجانب المقعّر من الكبد أخلاط نيئة. وإن كان مع الحمّى المحرقة بول رقيق فهو يدلّ على أنّ في العروق التي في حدبة الكبد أخلاطا نجّة كثيرة. في الثانية من شرحه لثالثة أبيديميا.

٤٦. الأعراض المقوّمة للحمّى المحرقة اثنان: العطش الدائم الذي لا ينقضي ولا يسكن والتهاب الحرارة التي تكون معها إحراق يدرك باللمس. في الثالثة من شرحه لثالثة أبيديميا.

٤٧. متى كانت القوى الثلاث كلّها قويّة والحمّى محرقة جدّا وتبيّنت علامات النضج ظاهرة فينبغي لك أن تسقي المريض ماء باردا بثقة واتّكال إلّا أن يكون شيخا هرما. ثانية عشر الحيلة.

٤٨. تولّد الحمّى المحرقة من عفن المرار الأصفر في المعدة وبخاصّة في فمها أو في مقعّر الكبد لا في أيّ عضو اتّفق. وأخصّ خواصّ الحمّى المحرقة أن يأتي بحرانها برعاف لأنّ الدم يعلو ويترقّى إلى فوق وتنبثق العروق. في الأولى من شرحه لأولى أبيديميا.

٤٩. الحمّيات المحرقة تتولّد إمّا من المرار الأصفر وإمّا عن البلغم المالح. في شرحه لثالثة الأمراض الحادّة.

---

٢ في] om. LOU || ٣ الحالين] الخلتين L || ٤ أبيديميا] أفيديميا LO: أبيديميا B || ٥ نيء] نيّ B || ٧ فهو] هو LOU || ٨ أبيديميا] أفيديميا LO || ١٠ إحراق] إندا L || ١١ أبيديميا] أفيديميا LO || ١٧ يعلو] يغلي GB | أبيديميا] أفيديميا ELO

(50) When a patient craves inhaling cold air because he has the sensation of a severe burning in the inner parts of his body, yet needs many clothes [to warm his body] from the outside because of the cold he feels, it is a sign that his illness is fatal, unless it occurs in the beginning of the [fever] attacks.[81] *In Hippocratis Epidemiarum* 2.3.[82]

(51) When the weather is cold, and [yet] the patient has [the sensation of] a severe burning, let your hope [that he will recover] be slim. If there are no clear signs of coction and he does not have much strength, it is impossible that he will escape [death]. *De methodo [medendi]* 11.[83]

(52) We apply clysters with olive oil and water only in ardent, burning fevers, in order to break their blazing and burning heat. *De clysteribus.*[84]

(53) In phlegmatic fevers the cause of rigor is not the same as the cause of the fever. The cause of the fever is that part of the phlegm that [has] putrefied, while the cause of the rigor is the remaining part of the phlegm, which has not yet putrefied. But in tertian fever, it is the yellow bile that produces both the rigor and the fever. *De [differentiis] febrium* 2.[85]

(54) With any illness that flares up and attacks in cycles, the cause[s] of its flaring up [in cycles] are the conditions of the organs [that occur in a certain order], whether it be the expulsion of the superfluities, or their acceptance, or their production and attraction. All this occurs because of a bad temperament of that organ—or of the [other] organs— that so weakens it that it accepts that which is expelled to it from another organ or attracts or alters that which is within it and produces superfluities. The organ that produces superfluities produces and expels them in cycles. Sometimes those superfluities remain within [the organ] until they putrefy. *De [differentiis] febrium* 2.[86]

Any illness that does not have cycles, such as continuous fever, is not caused by something specific for an organ of the body. But the humors in all the vessels, pulsatile and nonpulsatile—and especially those humors

٥٠. متى كان المريض يشتاق إلى استنشاق الهواء البارد لأنه يحسّ في أعضائه الباطنة بتلهّب شديد ويحتاج إلى دثار كثير لبرد يحسّه فذلك دليل على أنّ مرضه قتال إذا لم يكن ذلك في مبدأ النوائب. في ثالثة من شرحه لثانية أبيديميا.

٥١. إذا كان الهواء باردا والمريض يحترق احتراقا شديدا فليقلّ طمعك فيه. فإن لم تتبيّن فيه علامات النضج وكانت قوته ليست بالقوية فلا يمكن أن يفلت. حادية عشر الحيلة.

٥٢. نحن نحقن بالزيت والماء وحده في الحمّيات المحرقة الملتهبة لنكسر حرّ ذلك اللهيب والحرقة. في مقالته في الحقن.

٥٣. الحمّيات البلغمية سبب النافض فيها غير سبب الحمّى إذ سبب الحمّى هو الشيء الذي قد عفن من البلغم وسبب النافض هو الشيء الباقي من البلغم الذي لم يعفن بعد. فأمّا في حمّى الغبّ فإنّ المرّة الصفراء هي المحدثة للنافض والحمّى. في ثانية الحمّيات.

٥٤. كلّ ما كان من الأمراض يهيج وينوب على الأدوار فالسبب في هيجانه حالات راتبة في الأعضاء إمّا لأنها تدفع الفضول وإمّا لأنها تقبلها وإمّا لأنها تولّدها وإمّا لأنها تجذبها. كلّ ذلك من أجل سوء مزاج ذلك العضو أو الأعضاء الموجب لضعف قوته حتّى يقبل ما يدفع إليه غيره أو يجذب أو يحيل ما فيه ويولّد فضولا. فالعضو الذي يولّد الفضول قد يولّدها ويدفعها بأدوار. وقد تبقى فيه تلك الفضول حتّى تعفن. في ثانية الحمّيات.

ما كان من الأمراض ليس له أدوار كالحمّى الدائمة فليس سببه علّة خاصّة بعضو من أعضاء البدن، لكن الأخلاط التي في العروق كلّها الضوارب وغير الضوارب

---

in the largest and hottest vessels—become burning hot and boil because of putrefaction or for some other reason, as in the case of quotidian fever. This results in the development of one continuous, synochous fever from the beginning of the illness until its end. *De [differentiis] febrium* 2.[87]

(55) The decline and abatement of a fever attack refer to the entire time after the climax of the attack until the beginning of the next attack. *De crisibus* 1.[88]

(56) I have cured many people from quartan fever by administering the theriac, but first I emptied their bodies, then gave them absinthe juice to drink, and then this electuary two hours before the fever. The fever patient would be healed after two or three ingestions. *De theriaca ad Pisonem.*[89]

(57) Sometimes, in hectic fevers, the organ that becomes heated first is the heart. It is heated initially by an external cause: sometimes it is the liver, and sometimes the stomach, and after the stomach, the other organs that are capable of heating the heart until the hectic fever occurs. It is very beneficial to apply cooling remedies as soon as one observes signs of hectic fever in the organ that got heated first and that is the hearth of the fever. Similarly, marasmus occurring from hectic fevers should be treated with cooling substances taken internally, as well as applied externally to the painful organ. *De marcore liber.*[90]

(58) A specific, inseparable sign for anyone suffering from hectic fever is the following: when he takes food and waits for an hour, the heat of his body becomes inflamed and intense, but without oppression, and his pulse becomes greater and more rapid. Common to all hectic fevers is that the heat is always equally weak and feeble from its very beginning until its very end. One of the most important signs of hectic fevers is that the pulsatile vessels are found to be warmer than what surrounds them. *De febribus* 1.[91]

وخاصّة ماكان منها في أعظم العروق وأسخنها يلتهب ويغلي إمّا بسبب عفونة أو غيرها مثلحتى يوم فتتولّد حتى واحدة متصلة مطبقة من أوّل المرض إلى آخره. في ثانية الحمّيات.

٥٥. انحطاط نوبة الحمّى وسكونها هوجميع الوقت الذي بعد منتهى النوبة إلى ابتداء النوبة التالية لها. أولى البحران.

٥٦. قدأبرأت عدّة أناس من حمّى الربع بشرب الترياق إلا أنّي كنت أنفض أبدانهم أوّلا ثمّ أسقيهم عصارة الأفسنتين ثمّ من بعدها سقيتهم هذا المعجون قبل وقت الحمّى بساعتين. فكان المحموم يبرأ بشربتين أو بثلاث. في مقالته في الترياق إلى قيسر.

٥٧. قد يكون العضو الذي يسخن أوّلا في حمّيات الدقّ القلب. ويكون ابتداء سخونته من سبب من خارج، وقد يكون الكبد وقد تكون المعدة وبعد المعدة سائر الأعضاء التي يمكنها أن تسخن القلب حتّى يحدث الدقّ. ووضع الأدوية المبرّدة في أوّل ما تظهر علامات الدقّ على العضو الذي سخن أوّلا الذي هومستوقد الحمّى نافع جدّا. وكذلك الذبول الكائن من الحمّيات المحرقة برووءه يلتأم بالأشياء المبرّدة المستعملة من داخل والموضوعة على العضو الآلم من خارج. في مقالته في الذبول.

٥٨. أمرخاصّ غير مفارق لجميع من به حمّى الدقّ أن يكون إذا تناول الغذاء وأبطأ ساعة تلتهب حرارة بدنه وتقوى من غير تضاغط ويتزيّد نبضه عظما وسرعة. ويعمّ جميع حمّيات الدقّ أن تكون الحرارة ضعيفة رقيقة مستوية دائما منذ أوّل ابتدائها إلى آخرانقضائها. ومن أعظم دلائل حمّيات الدقّ أن توجد العروق الضاربة أسخن ممّا حولها. في أولى الحمّيات.

---

٤ الوقت...إلى آخره (٦٥) [om. O | إلى ابتداء النوبة [om. G || ٥ النوبة [om. E || ٨ بثلاث [ثلاث EL

(59) When the fever is accompanied by a diarrhea of liquified material, it is a pestilential fever, because this is an inseparable symptom of pestilential fever. *In Hippocratis Epidemiarum* 3.3.[92]

(60) We mostly find that hectic and marasmic fevers occur if the affliction [first] befell the heart, then the liver, and then the stomach. These fevers can also occur because of a hot and dry bad temperament that dominates the lungs, or the chest, or the mesentery. They can also occur because of an affliction befalling one of the intestines, or the uterus, or the kidneys, and then spreading to the substance of the heart. As for an affliction befalling the diaphragm first, I once saw hectic fever developing from an affliction occurring to it. But I do not know that I [ever] saw[93] marasmic fever developing from the diaphragm, because the patient would die before getting marasmus. *De methodo [medendi]* 10.[94]

(61) If someone has survived [an attack] of marasmic fever, then the marasmus occurred [only] in the flesh and similar structures. If the main organs[95] dry out, it is impossible that he should recover in any way. *De methodo [medendi]* 10.[96]

(62) All marasmic fevers belong to the type of fevers that cause the body to waste.[97] The difference between the two is that, in the case of marasmic fevers, the material that is wasted from the flesh is always eliminated through the pores, whereas in the case of [other] fevers that cause the body to waste, this material streams to the abdomen and is excreted in the stool. If this lasts for a long time, [as] in the case of someone who suffers from wasting fever but does not die, he develops marasmus. *De methodo [medendi]* 10.[98]

(63) The greatest and most effective means for treating continuous fevers are bloodletting—as much as the strength [of the patient] can tolerate—and the drinking of cold water after the coction [of the humors] (when the fever is of the type that develops from putrefaction). We have often observed that people who suffered from ardent fever drank cold water after the moderate coction of their humors, and the fever left them as soon as they drank it. *De methodo [medendi]* 9.[99]

٥٩. إذا كان مع الحمّى اختلاف شيء من جنس ما يذوب فتلك حمّى وبائية لأنّ هذا عرض لا يفارق الحمّى الوبائية. في ثالثة شرحه لثالثة أبيديميا.

٦٠. أكثر ما نجد حمّيات الدقّ وحمّيات الذبول تحدث إذا كانت الآفة إنّما نزلت بالقلب وبعده الكبد وبعدها المعدة. وقد تحدث أيضا من سوء مزاج حارّ يابس استولى على الرئة والصدر أو الماساريقا. وقد تحدث هذه الحمّى لآفة نزلت بأحد الأمعاء أو الأرحام أو الكليتين ويتعدّى ذلك إلى جرم القلب. وأمّا إن كانت الآفة نزلت أوّلا بالحجاب فقد رأيت مرّة حمّى دقّ حدثت عن الحجاب. وأمّا حمّى الذبول فلا أعلم أنّي رأيتها حدثت عن الحجاب إذا كان المريض يموت قبل أن ينتهي إلى الذبول. عاشرة الحيلة.

٦١. كلّ من ينجو من أصحاب الذبولية فإنّ الذبول كان في اللحم وما جانسه. فأمّا إن كانت الأعضاء الأصلية يبست فليس يمكن أن يبرأ بوجه. عاشر الحيلة.

٦٢. كلّ الحمّيات الذبولية داخلة في جنس الحمّيات التي تذيب البدن. والفرق بينها أنّ الشيء الذي يذوب من اللحم دائما يتحلّل من المسامّ في الحمّيات الذبولية ويجري ذلك ويسيل إلى البطن ويخرج في البراز في الحمّيات التي تذيب البدن. فإذا طال الأمر بأصحاب الحمّى الذبولية ولم يمت وقع إلى الذبول. عاشر الحيلة.

٦٣. أعظم الأشياء التي تعالج بها الحمّيات المطبقة وأبلغه الفصد حسب احتمال القوة وشرب الماء البارد بعد النضج إن كانت الحمّى من الصنف الكائن عن العفونة. وقد رأينا مرارا كثيرة قوما ممّن به حمّى محرقة قد شربوا الماء البارد بعد أن نضجت أخلاطهم نضجا معتدلا فأقلعت عنهم الحمّى ساعة شربوه. تاسعة الحيلة.

١ لأنّ هذا عرض لا يفارق الحمّى الوبائية] om. L || ٢ أبيديميا] أفيديميا ELO || ٤ نزلت] لزمت ELU || من] من أجل add. ELU || ٦ إلى جرم القلب] لجرم القلب ELU : لقلب B || ١٠ ينجو] يرجو L || ١١ عاشرة الحيلة] عاشر الحيلة EL || في تلك المقالة U || ١٥ عاشر الحيلة] عاشرة الحيلة EL || في تلك المقالة U || ١٦ وأبلغه] om. EL

If someone suffering from synochous fever falls into the hands of an ignorant physician who does not bleed the patient, then, by abstaining from bleeding him, he lets the fever increase and grow. Moreover, he shuts off all other avenues of treatment. For if he cools [him] down, he
5   destroys [him][100] because cooling, although it extinguishes the heat and balances the temperament, retains and keeps the overfilling within the body and prevents it from dissolving. But if he starts to evacuate the body with those things that are used to evacuate the body—and that are, all of them, hot—he will increase the heat of the fever. If someone neglects
10   bloodletting, he will eventually end up in this perplexing situation. *De methodo [medendi]* 9.[101]

(64) In all types of synochous fevers one should hasten to bleed the median cubital vein even to the point that the patient nearly faints, if his strength permits this. If someone suffering from this fever is not
15   bled from a vein, he falls into the greatest distress and is on the verge of the most extreme danger, unless he is saved from this by a strong nosebleed or profuse sweating. *De methodo [medendi]* 9.[102]

(65) There are two types of synochous—meaning continuous—fever. One type results from an obstruction occurring in the pores of the body
20   and is not accompanied by putrefaction of the humors. This synochous fever belongs to the genus of ephemeral fevers. Another type is that in which the obstruction is accompanied by the putrefaction of the humors, and it belongs to the genus of putrid fevers. Each one of these two types lasts for many days and constitutes a single attack from the beginning of
25   the illness until its end. In both types, one finds that the fever remains in the same state until the climax, that it increases little by little, and that it diminishes little by little. All of this depends upon the matter that burns up and the matter that dissolves from that which burns up. *De methodo [medendi]* 9.[103]

30   (66) The ephemeral fever that originates from an obstruction is sometimes so slow to abate that it seems as if it is not an ephemeral fever. In this case, one should apply venesection and extract blood in a quantity dependent on the strength [of the patient] and on the lightness or severity of the obstruction. The more severe the obstruction, the stronger
35   and shorter the fever. One should apply venesection] even if no signs of

متى وقعت حمّى سونوخس ليد طبيب جاهل فلم يفصد صاحبها فإنه إن ترك الفصد يزيدها وينميها. وتعطل سائر أبواب العلاج لأنه إن برّد أهلك لأنّ التبريد وإن كان يطفئ الحرارة ويعدّل المزاج فإنه يحقن ويحبس الامتلاء في جوف البدن ويمنع التحلّل. وإن أخذنا أن يستفرغ بالأشياء التي تستفرغ البدن كلّها حارّة فيزيد في حرارة

٥ الحمّى. فمن أهمل الفصد وصل به الأمر أخيرا إلى هذه الحيرة. تاسعة الحيلة.

٦٤. جميع أصناف حمّيات سونوخس يجب أن تبادر فيها بفصد الأكحل حتّى يقارب العليل الغشي إن ساعدت القوة. ومتى لم تقصد لصاحب هذه الحمّى عرقا وقع إلى غاية البلاء وأشرف على نهاية الخطر إلا أن يتخلّص من ذلك برعاف شديد أو بعرق عزيز. تاسعة الحيلة.

٦٥. حمّى سونوخس وهي الحمّى المطبقة صنفان. صنف يتولّد عن سدد تحدث

١٠ في مسامّ البدن ولا تحدث معه عفونة في الأخلاط. وهذه هي حمّى سونوخس التي هي جنس من حمّى يوم. ومنها صنف تعفن فيه الأخلاط مع تلك السدد وهو من جنس حمّى العفونة. وكلّ واحد من هذين الصنفين يدوم أيّاما كثيرة وهي نوبة واحدة من أوّل المرض إلى آخره. فمن الصنفين جميعا ما يدوم على حالة واحدة إلى وقت المنتهى ومنها ما يزيد أوّلا أوّلا ومنها ما ينقص أوّلا أوّلا. وكلّ ذلك بحسب

١٥ الشيء المحترق والشيء الذي يتحلّل ممّا احترق. تاسعة الحيلة.

٦٦. حمّى اليوم الحادثة عن السدد قد يبطئ انحطاطها حتّى يتخيّل أنّها ليست حمّى يوم. وينبغي أن تقصد فيها العرق ويخرج الدم بحسب القوة وبحسب كثرة السدد وقلّتها. وكلّ ما كانت السدد أكثر كانت الحمّى أقوى وأقصر ولو لم تكن علامات

---

١ إن ترك] بترك ELBU || ٥ فن] فإن ELB || ٩ تاسعة الحيلة] في تلك مقالة EL || ١٠ سونوخس] سنوخس EL صنفان] منها add ELBU عن] من EL || ١١ سونوخس] سنوخس L: سونوخس E || ١٢ من حمّى يوم] om. ELU

overfilling occur together [with the fever]. For then the gaseous superfluity diminishes through the decrease in humors, and opening the
obstruction will be easier afterwards. After the bleeding, treat the
patient with oxymel and then with barley gruel. If you see, on the third
day, that only a small amount of fever remains and that there are no
clear signs of putrefaction, neither in the urine nor in the pulse, let him
go to the bathhouse three or four hours prior to the time that you expect
[another fever] attack. *De methodo [medendi]* 8.[104]

(67) No fever develops from an indigestion in which the food turns
sour. But fever can occur from an indigestion in which the food becomes
gaseous. If someone develops a fever from such an indigestion and also
suffers from diarrhea, and if you see that the evacuated matter consists
only of that which was corrupted, let the patient bathe and feed him
during the abatement of the first attack and take care to strengthen his
stomach. But if you see that the earlier or later[105] evacuation was so
extreme that it wears out the strength [of the patient], the best thing
[to do] is to feed him without having him go to the bathhouse. *De methodo [medendi]* 8.[106]

(68) Food [intake] is the worst thing for anyone whose fever is
caused by overfilling, or an obstruction, or an [inflamed] tumor, or
putrefaction of the humors. Do not feed them—not even when the
[fever] attack abates. For anyone whose fever is caused by sleeplessness
or worry or anxiety or emotions, abstention from food is the worst. One
may feed them at any time during the attack of the fever, but especially
when it abates. *De methodo [medendi]* 10.[107]

(69) Someone suffering from continuous fever should be nourished
at such time that he feels at ease and [better], and especially at the
time that he was accustomed to eating when he was healthy. *De methodo
[medendi]* 11.[108]

(70) One should evacuate the putrid superfluities from patients with
continuous fever by prescribing diuretics and purgatives, by stimulating
perspiration, and by inducing emesis when these superfluities spontane-
ously move toward the stomach. But if they do not move toward the

الا متلاء مجتمعة ليقلّ الفضل الدخاني بقلّة الأخلاط ويسهل تفتيح السدد بعد ذلك.
وبعد فصد تداويه بالسكنجبين وبعده بماء كشك الشعير. وإذا رأيت أنّ الذي بقي من
الحمّى في اليوم الثالث شيء يسير ولم تتبيّن علامات عفونة لا في البول ولا في النبض
فأدخله الحمّام قبل وقت توقع النوبة بثلاث ساعات أو أربع. ثامنة الحيلة.

٦٧. التخمة التي يستحيل الطعام فيها إلى حموضة ليس تحدث عنها حمّى. وإنّما يمكن
حدوث الحمّى عن التخمة التي يستحيل فيها الطعام إلى الدخانية. فمن حمّ من تلك التخمة
وانطلق طبعه معها فإن رأيت أنّ الذي استفرغ إنّما هو الشيء الذي قد فسد فقط
فأدخل المريض الحمّام وغذه عند انحطاط النوبة الأولى وتعني بتقوية معدته. وإن
رأيت أنّ الذي تقدّم استفراغه أو الشيء الحاضر قد أفرط إلى أن أجحف بالقوة
فالأجود أن تغذوه من غير أن تدخله الحمّام. ثامنة الحيلة.

٦٨. كلّ من حمّاه بسبب امتلاء أو بسبب سدد أو بسبب ورم أو بسبب
عفونة الأخلاط فإنّ الطعام أردأ ما يكون لهم ولا تغذوهم ولو في انحطاط النوبة.
وكلّ من حمّاه من أجل سهر أو غمّ أو وهم أو انفعالات نفسانية فالإمساك عن الطعام
أضرّ شيء لهم. وتقدر أن تغذوهم في كلّ أوقات النوبة وبخاصّة في انحطاطها.
عاشر الحيلة.

٦٩. يكون وقت تغذية المريض في الحمّيات المطبقة في الوقت الذي يجد فيه راحة
ويحسّ بخفة وخاصّة وقت عادته في حال صحته. حادية عشر الحيلة.

٧٠. ينبغي أن تستفرغ الفضول العفنة من أصحاب الحمّيات المطبقة بإدرار البول
وبإسهال البطن وبإدرار العرق وباستدعاء القيء إن تحرّكت الفضول نحو المعدة من

___

٢ رأيت] كانت O | أنّ] كانت O | ٧ الذي] G¹ | om. ELOU | ٩ أنّ] om. ELBOU ||
١٠ ثامنة الحيلة] في تلك المقالة ELO | ١٧ بخفة] بحفّ ELBOU | ١٩ من تلقاء
أنفسها. أمّا إن لم تتحرّك إلى المعدة] G¹

stomach, do not induce emesis; rather, choose those remedies by which such an evacuation can be effected without producing heat [at all] or [producing] only a minor amount of heat. *De methodo [medendi]* 11.[109]

(71) To feed someone suffering from [inflamed] tumors in the liver or stomach before a [fever] attack is one of the most destructive and fatal things for him. When the liver or stomach is weak but without [inflamed] tumors, to do so is one of the most beneficial things. *De methodo [medendi]* 11.[110]

This is the end of the tenth treatise,
by the grace of God, praise be to Him.

◆

تلقاء أنفسها. أمّا إن لم تتحرّك إلى المعدة فلا تستدعي القيء، وتقصد من الأدوية التي تفعل بها أحد هذه الاستفراغات ما لا يسخن أو يسخن إسخانا يسيرا. حادية عشر الحيلة.

٧١. متى كانت الكبد أو المعدة وارمة فالتغذية قبل النوبة من أهلك الأشياء وأقتلها للمريض. وإن كانت الكبد أو المعدة ضعيفة من غير ورم فذلك من أنفع الأشياء. حادية عشر الحيلة.

تمّت المقالة العاشرة ولله الحمد والمنة.

---

٧ تمت المقالة العاشرة ولله الحمد والمنة] om. O : تمت المقالة العاشرة والحمد لله وعدد فصولها ثلاثة وسبعون فصلا L : كملت المقالة العاشرة وعدد فصولها ثلاثة وسبعون فصلا والحمد لله ⟨ . . . ⟩ E : تمت المقالة العاشرة B : تمت المقالة الثانية والحمد لله وعدد فصولها أربعة وسبعين U

In the name of God,
the Merciful, the Compassionate.
O Lord, make [our task] easy

The Eleventh Treatise

Containing aphorisms concerning
the periods and crisis of a disease

(1) The periods of a disease are four altogether: beginning, increase, culmination and decline. It is only with great toil that one can come to know the actual period of a disease at a certain moment through an exact conjecture.[1] *De crisibus* 1.[2]

(2) We find that [in the case of] the disease which is extremely grave—namely, apoplexy—its beginning and increase take place in a short time. The same holds true for epilepsy,[3] for it does not occur in the same way as that which happens to those whose head is cut off, although [even here] the beheading takes a first and a second and a third time.[4] And when we admit that epilepsy and apoplexy occur without taking time, we mean the symptoms that follow these diseases; while the disease itself that causes apoplexy and epilepsy has, without any doubt, the four periods.[5] *De [totius] morbi temporibus.*[6]

بسم الله الرحمن الرحيم

رب يسّر

المقالة الحادية العشر

تشتمل على فصول تتعلّق

بأوقات المرض وبحرانه

٥

١. أوقات المرض الكلّية أربعة: ابتداء وتزيّد وانتهاء وانحطاط. وبكدّ ما يوقف على معرفة الوقت الحاضر من أوقات المرض بحدس صحيح أيّ أوقاته هو الآن. أولى البحران.

٢. نجد المرض الذي يكون في غاية الشدّة وهو السكتة ابتداءه وصعوده في مدّة قصيرة. وكذلك الصرع فإنّه لا يحدث كمن يضرب عنقه على أن ضرب العنق

١٠ له وقت أوّل وثاني وثالث. فإن سامحنا في أنّ حدوث الصرع والسكتة بلا زمان فهما أعراض تابعة لأمراض والمرض الموجب للسكتة والصرع له بلا شكّ الأوقات الأربعة. في مقالته في أوقات المرض.

---

(3) The time of the beginning of a disease is [measured] from its first minute until [signs of] coction [of the corrupt matter] begin to appear. When the coction increases and the disease worsens, all this is the time of the increase, until the disease is as severe as possible; and this is the time of the climax. Any crisis comes only during the time of the climax of the disease, and the time of the entire crisis is the time of the climax. After the climax begins the decline, until the patient is cured. *De crisibus* 1.[7]

(4) In some diseases the time of the occurrence of a disease—that is, the time of its beginning—as well as the time of its increase, are hidden from the senses. But the time of the climax can be perceived in all diseases. If a particular patient is likely to be cured from his disease, this time is followed by a perceptible decline. Thus, it is clear that, in a number of diseases, neither the beginning nor the increase is perceptible. *De morborum temporibus.*[8]

(5) Sometimes a hard tumor occurs on the concave side of the liver and persists for a long time, while it is hidden from our senses, and the passage of food becomes spoiled, while we do not know at what time this occurs. With the passage of time, dropsy develops, whereby one assumes that the disease is, at that actual moment, in [the phase] of beginning or increase. I have seen a similar thing occurring to many people. *De morborum temporibus.*[9]

(6) Sometimes the first fever attack covers the beginning, increase, and climax of the disease, so that the beginning of the attack is the beginning of the disease, the increase [of the disease] is the following phase of the attack, and the climax [of the disease] falls together with the climax of the attack. Then, in the second [fever] attack, the signs of the decline [of the disease] become clearly perceptible. *De crisibus* 1.[10]

٣. زمان الابتداء هو من أوّل دقيقة من المرض إلى أن يبتدئ ظهور النضج. ومنذ يأخذ النضج في الزيادة والمرض يتزيّد شدّة فهذا كلّه زمان التزيّد حتّى يصل المرض إلى أشدّ ما يكون هو زمان المنتهى. وكلّ بحران إنّما يأتي في وقت منتهى المرض وزمان البحران كلّه هو زمان المنتهى. وبعد المنتهى يبتدئ الانحطاط إلى أن ٥ ينقه المريض. أولى البحران.

٤. وقت حدوث المرض وهو زمان الابتداء وكذلك وقت التزيّد قد يخفى عن الحسّ في بعض الأمراض. فأمّا زمان المنتهى محسوس في جميع الأمراض. فإن كان من شأن هذا المريض أن يتخلّص من مرضه أعقب هذا الوقت انحطاط محسوس. فقد بان أن ثمّ عدّة أمراض لا يحسّ فيها بابتداء ولا بتزيّد. في مقالته في أوقات الأمراض.

٥. قد يمكن أن يحدث في الجانب المقعّر من الكبد ورم منفجّر فيدوم مدّة من الزمان ١٠ وهو خفيّ عن حسّنا. فيفسد نفوذ الغذاء من غير أن يمكننا معرفة ذلك الوقت. وإذا طال الزمان عرض الاستسقاء فيظنّ به أنّه الآن ابتداء وتزيّد. وقد رأيت خلقا كثيرا عرض لهم مثل هذه الحال. في مقالته في أوقات الأمراض.

٦. ربّما اشتملت النوبة الأولى من الحمّى على ابتداء المرض وتزيّده ومنتهاه حتّى ١٥ يكون أوّل النوبة هو أوّل المرض وتزيّده في ما يتلو ذلك وانتهاه مع انتهاء النوبة. ثمّ تظهر في النوبة الثانية علامات الانحطاط ظهورا بيّنا. أولى البحران.

---

٢ ومنذ يأخذ النضج] om. ELOU || ٣ وكلّ... كلّه هو زمان المنتهى] om. B | وقت] om. ELOU || ٥ أولى البحران] G¹ || ٧ فأمّا زمان المنتهى محسوس في جميع الأمراض] om. ELU || ١١ من] om. G | يمكننا] om. ELOU | الوقت] om. ELU | الوقت] عسر G¹ || ١٢ الآن] om. ELU || ١٥ وتزيّده] add. ELU | ومنتهاه] add. G

(7) The end of the time of the beginning [of a disease]—that is, the beginning of the time of its increase—is [marked by] the appearance of a clear sign indicating coction. A clear sign holds the middle between hidden, weak signs[11] of coction and signs of complete coction. *De crisibus* 1.[12]

(8) A sign[13] of complete coction is that a white, even, and smooth sediment appears in the urine. A sign of weak coction is when the color of the urine changes from that of water to pale yellow, or that it changes from a clear condition into a turbid one. Similarly, when the urine has a fine consistency and is bright[14] [yellowish red], it is a weak sign. In the case of all these weak signs, the disease is in its beginning. *De crisibus* 1.[15]

(9) A sign that clearly indicates that the beginning of the disease has come to an end is the appearance of a white, even, and continuous cloud [in the urine], either suspended in its middle or floating upon it. Similarly, a deep red cloud [in the urine], or a deep red sediment, or urine that is moderately thick [and] has a healthy color but no sediment is a clear sign indicating the beginning of the increase [of the disease].[16] *De crisibus* 1.[17]

(10) The quick end of a disease which comes with great strain and which is called by the special name "crisis" is especially characteristic of fevers that originate from hot chymes. Moreover, it is found in the case of inflamed tumors that are quick to move[18] in the major organs. *De crisibus* 2.[19]

(11) If the illness is severe and strong, it inevitably ends with a crisis. But when it is small and weak, its end does not come with a crisis. A crisis always comes on a day of attack [of the illness]. It only rarely comes on a day that it is quiescent. I have seen such an exceptional [case] only once. *De crisibus* 3.[20]

٧. آخر زمان الابتداء وهو ابتداء زمان التزيّد هو ظهور علامة بيّنة تدلّ على النضج. والعلامة البيّنة هي بين علامات النضج الخفية الضعيفة وبين علامات النضج التامّ. أولى البحران.

٨. علامات النضج التامّ هي أن يظهر في البول ثفل راسب أبيض مستوٍ ٥ أملس. وعلامات النضج الخفية هي انتقال البول عن لون الماء إلى أن يضرب للصفرة قليلا أو أن ينتقل عن حال الرقة إلى الخثورة. وكذلك البول الدقيق القوام المشبع هو أيضا علامة خفية. ومع هذه الخفية كلّها فالمرض في ابتدائه. أولى البحران.

٩. العلامات البيّنة التي تدلّ على أنّ ابتداء المرض قد انقضى هي ظهور غمامة بيضاء مستوية متصلة إمّا متعلّقة في وسطه أو طافية عليه. وكذلك الغمامة التي ١٠ لونها أحمر قانئ والثفل الراسب الأحمر القانئ وكذلك البول الحسن اللون المعتدل اللّون علامة بيّنة تدلّ على ابتداء التزيّد وعلى أنّ لا ثفل فيه. أولى البحران.

١٠. انقضاء المرض الحثيث الذي يكون معه جهد عظيم وهو الذي يسمّى خاصّة باسم البحران إنّما هو خاص بالحمّيات المتولّدة من الكيموسات الحارة. ثمّ بعد ذلك فهو يوجد للأورام الحارّة السريعة الحركة التي تكون في أعضاء ذات خطر. ١٥ ثانية البحران.

١١. إن كان المرض عظيما قويا كان انقضاؤه لا محالة بحران. وإن كان يسيرا ضعيفا كان انقضاؤه لا بحران. والبحران أبدا في يوم النوبة وأمّا مجيء البحران في يوم الراحة فلا يكاد يكون إلا في الندرة وإلى هذه الغاية لم أره إلا مرة واحدة. ثالثة البحران.

---

٢ بين] om. G | وبين] G || ٦ الخثورة] الخثرة ELO: الخثور U: الخثير B || ٧ هذه الخفية كلّها] هذا الخفا كلّه L || ٨ هي] هو L || ١٢ الحثيث] الحاذ L: الحديث O || ١٣ خاصّ] G¹ || ١٦ وإن كان يسيرا ضعيفا كان انقضا ٥ لا بحران] om. ELO

(12) Complete coction occurs especially during the climax of a disease. A salutary crisis comes during the climax or shortly before it. The crisis that is closer to the climax is always more salutary than the one that is more distant from it. Once complete coction has become evident, it is impossible that a nonsalutary crisis occur at any time. *De crisibus* 3.[21]

(13) There are five signs that indicate that a current crisis is beneficial: The first and the most important is that the coction comes first. I have never seen anyone die as a result of a crisis coming to him after coction. The second sign is that it [i.e., the coction] occurs on one of the days of the crisis. The third sign is that the crisis is announced beforehand on a day bordering on the crisis.[22] The fourth sign is that the crisis is light and easy. The fifth sign is that the evacuation is congenial to the nature and way[23] of the disease. *De crisibus* 3.[24]

(14) Perspiration is congenial to[25] all fevers, especially those that are severely burning and ardent. A nosebleed is congenial to all inflamed internal tumors,[26] except for an [inflamed] tumor on the concave side of the liver, because diarrhea, perspiration, or emesis are congenial to its crisis. The same holds good for diseases of the chest and lungs, for expectoration is congenial to their crisis. *De crisibus* 3.[27]

(15) In the case of diseases of the head, a certainly safe crisis is sometimes brought about through tumors appearing at the roots of the ears;[28] and in the case of chronic fevers, through tumors and abscesses[29] appearing in other parts of the body. *De crisibus* 3.[30]

(16) The signs which indicate that the next crisis will be bad are not reliable and accurate, especially since a crisis may occur that does not necessarily follow from such signs.[31] The signs which indicate that the next crisis is salutary are reliable and accurate[32] and are [therefore] followed by a salutary crisis, according to their indication. *De crisibus* 3.[33]

١٢.   النضج المستحكم إنما يكون في منتهى المرض. والبحران المحمود يأتي عند المنتهى أو قبله بقليل. والبحران أبدا الأقرب من المنتهى أحمد من البحران الأبعد منه. وليس يمكن بعد ظهور النضج المستحكم أن يأتي في الوقت من الأوقات بحران غير محمود. ثالثة البحران.

١٣.   العلامات الدالّة على جودة البحران الحاضرة خمسة: أوّلها وأعظمها تقدّم النضج ولم أر أحدا قط مات ممّن أتاه البحران بعد النضج. الثانية أن يكون في يوم من أيام البحران. الثالث أن يتقدّمه إنذار في يوم مواصل له. الرابعة أن يكون البحران سهلا خفيفا. الخامسة أن يكون الاستفراغ مشاكلا لطبيعة المرض وجهته. ثالثة البحران.

١٤.   العرق يشاكل جميع الحمّيات وبخاصة ماكان منها شديد الالتهاب محرقا. والرعاف يشاكل جميع الأورام الحارّة الباطنة إلا أن يكون الورم في مقعّر الكبد فإنّ بحرانه المشاكل اختلاف أو عرق أو قيء. وكذلك علل الصدر والرئة فإنّ بحرانه المشاكل بالنفث. ثالثة البحران.

١٥.   قد يكون بحران يوثق بصحّته في علل الرأس بأورام تظهر في أصل الأذنين وفي الحمّيات المتطاولة بأورام وخراجات تظهر في مواضع أخر من البدن. ثالثة البحران.

١٦.   الدلائل التي يستدلّ بها على أنّ البحران الذي يأتي يكون رديئا ليست بالصحيحة الثابتة، بل قد يأتي بحران غير لازم عن تلك العلامات. وأمّا الدلائل التي يستدلّ بها على أنّ البحران الذي يأتي محمودا فهي صحيحة ثابتة ويأتي بعدها بحران محمود كما دلّت. ثالثة البحران.

---

(17) Many times a person suffers from sleeplessness, heaviness of the head, indolence, lack of energy to move, lack of appetite, weariness, headache, and the like while he carries out his normal activities. But then these symptoms increase so much that they throw him down and he has to lie down. The beginning of his illness should be reckoned from that moment in which he clearly began to suffer from such a high fever that he was forced to lie down. *De diebus decretoriis* 1.[34]

(18) The most eminent and powerful critical day is the seventh. The fourth day is mostly announced by a clear change taking place on it, in either the urine, or sputum, or excrements, or appetite, or understanding, or sensation, or other things. The change that occurs on the seventh day always resembles that occurring on the fourth day. If the change on the fourth day is for the better, then the crisis on the seventh day is good; and if it is for the worse, then the crisis on the seventh day is bad. Most of those whose condition changes for the worse on the fourth day die on the sixth day. *De diebus decretoriis* 1.[35]

(19) The fourteenth [day] is closest[36] in its nature to the seventh. Similarly, the ninth, eleventh, and twentieth [days] are close to the nature of the fourteenth.[37] Next [in closeness] comes the fourth day, and then the third, fifth, and eighteenth.[38] *De diebus decretoriis* 1.[39]

(20) As for the other critical days after the twentieth until the fortieth day, critical movement is weaker in all of them and slowly becomes less.[40] And those that come after the fortieth day are very weak. During these critical days, the end of the illness [occurs] either through coction or through an abscess or, in rare cases, through evacuation. *De diebus decretoriis* 1.[41]

(21) I have never seen anyone to whom a crisis occurred on the twelfth and sixteenth day of the illness. Similarly, the nineteenth day is not a critical day; neither [is] the first nor the second day. On the sixth day, a crisis indeed occurs to some patients but is accompanied by severe symptoms and grave danger. It is not a true crisis and does not come to an end but leads to worse [symptoms]. *De diebus decretoriis* 1.[42]

١٧. كثيرًا ما يعرض للإنسان سهر وثقل رأس وكسل وقلة نشاط للحركة وقلة شهوة وإعياء وصداع وأشياء شبيهة بهذه وهو يتصرف على معتاده وتلك الأعراض تتزيّد حتّى تصرعه ويضطجع. فيعدّ أول المرض من ذلك الوقت الذي تبتدئ فيه الحمّى ابتداء ظاهرًا حتّى يضطرّ المريض إلى الاضطجاع. الأولى من أيّام البحران.

٥ ١٨. المتقدّم لجميع أيّام البحران في قوّته وشرفه هو اليوم السابع. وينذر به الرابع في أكثر الحالات بتغيّر بيّن يحدث فيه إمّا في البول أو في ما ينفث أو في البراز أو في الشهوة أو في الفهم أو الحسّ أو ما سوى ذلك. والتغيّر الحادث في السابع مشاكل أبدًا لما حدث في الرابع إن كان الذي حدث في الرابع إلى ما هو خير فبحران السابع يكون جيّدًا. وإن كان تغيّر الرابع إلى ما هو شرّ فبحران السابع يكون رديئًا. وأكثر من ١٠ يتغيّر حاله في الرابع إلى الشرّ يموتون في السادس. الأولى من أيّام البحران.

١٩. الرابع عشر قريب في طبيعته من اليوم السابع، وكذلك التاسع والحادي عشر والعشرون قريب من طبيعة الرابع عشر. ومن بعد هذه الرابع وبعد الرابع الثالث والخامس والثامن عشر. الأولى من أيّام البحران.

٢٠. سائر أيّام البحران التي بعد العشرين إلى الأربعين الحركة البحرانية فيها كلّها ضعيفة وتنقص قليلًا قليلًا. وأمّا التي بعد الأربعين فهي ضعيفة جدًا. وانقضاء المرض ١٥ فيها إمّا بالنضج أو بخراج وقلّ ما يكون باستفراغ. الأولى من أيّام البحران.

٢١. اليوم الثاني عشر من المرض واليوم السادس عشر منه لم أر أحدًا قطّ أصابه فيه بحران. وكذلك التاسع عشر ليس هو يوم بحران ولا اليوم الأوّل ولا الثاني. وأمّا اليوم السادس فقد يصيب بعض المرضى فيه بحران لكن مع أعراض صعبة وخطر ٢٠ شديد. وليس يصحّ بحرانه ولا يتمّ ويؤول إلى شرّ. الأولى من أيّام البحران.

٣ تصرعه] تضعه B ‖ ٤ فيه...بحران (٢٨)] om. L ‖ ٩ فبحران] فإنّ G ‖ ١٤ إلى] G¹ ‖ ١٦ البحران] G¹

(22) If a crisis happens to occur on the eighth or tenth [day], it is similar to the crisis that occurs on the sixth [day]. *De diebus decretoriis* 1.[43]

(23) When it is said of a crisis that it does not come to an end, it means a crisis in which the rest of the symptoms of the illness remain until after that crisis. When it is said of a crisis that it is not a true one,[44] it means a crisis after which the illness returns. A dangerous and incomplete crisis is the one which comes with severe symptoms, whereby one has to fear for the [life of] the patient. An unclear crisis is that in which there is no clear evacuation nor clear abscess. Sometimes a crisis comes suddenly, without previous announcement.[45] *De diebus decretoriis* 1.[46]

(24) An acute illness is one that moves fast and is dangerous. An illness that is very acute to the extreme[47] is one that ends on the fourth day. One that is very acute but not to the extreme is one which ends on the seventh. An absolutely acute[48] illness is the one that ends on the fourteenth day, and this is the one that is really acute. An illness that ends after the fourteenth day and before the twentieth day is somehow reckoned among the acute ones but is only called acute in a figurative sense. The illness occurring from a relapse is also called acute. *De diebus decretoriis* 1.[49]

(25) From three things, one can draw conclusions as to whether the periods of an illness will be long or short: from the nature of the illness, from the seasons of the year, and from the evacuations from the body. [Conclusions can be drawn] from the nature of an illness, as is the case in illnesses arising from black [bile] (such as quartan fever) and from phlegm (such as sciatica and pain in the kidneys and arthritis), since these have long beginnings and also remote [distant] culminations. But ardent fever, pleurisy, and pneumonia have short beginnings and near culminations.[50] The nearness of the culmination is according to the acuteness of the illness. One can conclude [the duration of periods] from the seasons of the year because all illnesses have shorter beginnings and more rapid endings in the summer and lengthier beginnings and slower

٢٢. إن اتّفق أن يعرض بحران في الثامن أو العاشر فهو شبيه البحران الذي يكون في السادس. الأولى من أيّام البحران.

٢٣. متى قيل بحران لم يتمّ فهو البحران الذي يبقى من أعراض المرض بقية بعد ذلك البحران. ومتى قيل بحران لم يصحّ فهو الذي يعاود المرض بعده. والبحران الخطر والغير

٥ سليم هو الذي تكون معه أعراض صعبة يخاف على المريض منها. والبحران الغير بيّن هو الذي لا يكون معه استفراغ بيّن ولا خراج ظاهر. وقد يأتي البحران بغتة ولا يتقدّمه إنذار. الأولى من أيّام البحران.

٢٤. المرض الحادّ هو الذي يتحرّك حركة سريعة وفيه خطر. والمرض الحادّ جدّا في الغاية هو الذي ينقضي في الرابع. والذي هو حادّ جدّا لا في الغاية هو الذي ينقضي في

١٠ السابع. والحادّ بقول مرسل هو الذي ينتهي إلى الرابع عشر وهو حادّ بالحقيقة. وأمّا ما ينقضي من بعد الرابع عشر إلى العشرين فإنّه ينسب إلى الحدّة نسبة ما ولا يقال له حادّ إلّا على المجاز. وقد يسمّى أيضا حادّا ما عرض من النكس. الأولى من أيّام البحران.

٢٥. يستدلّ على أوقات المرض هل هي طويلة أو قصيرة من ثلاثة أشياء: من طبيعة المرض ومن أوقات السنة وممّا يبرز من البدن. أمّا من طبيعة المرض

١٥ فكلّ أمراض الكائنة عن السوداء كالربع والبلغم ووجع النساء ووجع الكلى ووجع المفاصل فإنّ ابتداءها طويلا ومنتهاها أيضا بعيدا. وأمّا الحمّى المحرقة وذات الجنب وذات الرئة فابتداؤها قصير ومنتهاها قريب. وعلى حسب حدّة المرض يكون قرب منتهاه. وأمّا الاستدلال من أوقات السنة فإنّ جميع الأمراض يكون في الصيف أقصر ابتداء وأسرع انقضاء وفي الشتاء أطول ابتداء وأبطأ انقضاء. وأمّا

---

١ شبيه] يشبه EBOU || ٢ أيّام] G¹ || ١٧ حدّة] هذه OU

endings in the winter. One can conclude [duration] from the evacuations [from the body] because the appearance of good sputum, or similar urine or excrements, or perspiration in the beginning of the illness indicates that the beginning will be short and that the climax is near, while a delay in its appearance indicates that [the beginning] will be prolonged. *De crisibus* 1.[51]

(26) In some incomplete crises, such a large quantity of superfluities streams to a small organ that this organ cannot contain it. Then that superfluity returns to its [original] site or to a major organ, and the patient dies. *In Hippocratis Epidemiarum* 2.1.[52]

(27) The days of crisis are every fourth day[53] until the twentieth day: namely, the fourth, the seventh, the eleventh, the fourteenth, the seventeenth, and the twentieth. After the twentieth, they are every seventh day until the fortieth day. After the fortieth, they are computed in terms of every twentieth day until the hundred and twentieth day. After the hundred and twentieth day, one computes these days in terms of cycles of months, just like the cycles of days. And after the cycles of months, [one computes them] in terms of cycles of years. *In Hippocratis Epidemiarum* 2.1.[54]

(28) Illnesses that last longer than forty days hardly ever have a crisis through perspiration and definitely do not have a crisis through some [other] type of evacuation. But their end comes either through gradual coction or through an abscess. *In Hippocratis Aphorismos commentarius* 4.[55]

(29. In the case of continuous fevers, one should count [all] the successive days [for a prognosis of the future crisis]; but in the case of intermittent fevers, one should count only the days of their bouts. For the effect of the seventh day in the case of continuous fevers is similar to the effect of the seventh cycle in the case of tertian fevers. Similarly, in the case of pure quartan fever, a crisis comes in seven cycles, that is, [on] the nineteenth day. *In Hippocratis Prognostica commentarius* 3.[56]

الاستدلال مِمّا يبرز فإنّ ظهور النفث الحسن أو البول أو البراز الذي هو كذلك والعرق من أول المرض يدلّ على قصر الابتداء وقرب المنتهى وتأخّر ظهور هذه يدلّ على الطول. أولى البحران.

٢٦. قد ينصبّ في البحارين الناقصة فضل كثير إلى عضو صغير فلا يسعه ذلك العضو فيرجع الفضل إلى موضعه أو إلى عضو شريف فيقتل. في الأولى من شرحه لثانية أبيديميا.

٢٧. أيّام البحران أربعة إلى العشرين وهي الرابع والسابع والحادي عشر والرابع عشر والسابع عشر والعشرين. ومن بعد العشرين سبعة سبعة إلى الأربعين ويُحسب بعد الأربعين عشرين عشرين إلى المائة وعشرين. ويُحسب بعد المائة وعشرين على أدوار الشهور كأدوار الأيّام وبعد الشهور على أدوار السنين. في السادسة من شرحه لثانية أبيديميا.

٢٨. الأمراض التي تجاوز الأربعين يوما لا يكاد يكون فيها بحران بعرق ولا بنوع من أنواع الاستفراغ بتّة، لكن انقضاءها يكون إمّا بنضج أوّلا أوّلا أو بخراج. في شرحه لرابعة الفصول.

٢٩. احسب في الحمّيات الدائمة الأيّام على ولائها وفي الحمّيات التي لها نوائب أيّام نوائبها فقط لأنّ ما يفعله اليوم السابع في الحمّيات الدائمة يفعله الدور السابع في الحمّيات التي تنوب غبّا. وكذلك الربع الخالصة يأتي فيها بحران في سبعة أدوار وهو اليوم التاسع عشر. في شرحه لثالثة تقدمة المعرفة.

---

٦ أبيديميا] أفيديميا EOU ‖ ٨ ومن...إلى] G¹ ‖ ٩ بعد] ذلك add. U ‖ المائة] ذلك add. B ‖ ١١ أبيديميا] أفيديميا EOU

(30) From[57] six things, one can conclude that a crisis is complete and perfect. The first and the most important is that it is preceded by clear coction. The second is that it occurs through evacuation and not through an abscess. The third is that the evacuated matter consists of bad chyme. The fourth is that the evacuation is from the side of the illness. The fifth is that this is done on a critical day. The sixth is that it is followed by alleviation and total relaxation.[58] *In Hippocratis Aphorismos commentarius* 4.[59]

This is the end of the eleventh treatise,
by the grace of God, praise be to Him.

◆

٣٠. يستدلّ على أنّ البحران تامّ كامل بستّة أشياء: أوّلها وهو أعظمها أن يتقدّمه النضج البيّن. الثاني أن يكون باستفراغ لا بخراج. الثالث أن يكون الشيء المستفرغ كيموسا رديئا. الرابع أن يكون الاستفراغ من جانب المرض. الخامس أن يكون في يوم بحران. السادس أن يتبعه الخفّ والراحة الكاملة. في شرحه

٥ لأولى الفصول.

تمّت المقالة الحادي عشر ولله الحمد والمنّة.

---

٦ تمّت المقالة الحادي عشر ولله الحمد والمنّة [om. O : تمّت المقالة وعدد فصولها ثلاثون فصلا L : تمّت المقالة الحادية عشر والحمد لله كثيرا E : تمّت المقالة الحادية عشر B : تمّت المقالة الثالثة لحبيش والحمد لله عدد فصولها ثلاثون U

In the name of God,
the Merciful, the Compassionate.
O Lord, make [our task] easy

The Twelfth Treatise

5 *Containing aphorisms concerning*
evacuation by means of bloodletting

(1) From the following three things one can determine the necessity of venesection: severity of the current or expected illness; age [of the patient]—that he is not too old nor too young—and great strength. *De venae sectione.*[1]

(2) If someone has broad and large [nonpulsatile] vessels and his body is somewhat lean and his complexion is not white and his flesh is not soft, one should bleed him without caution and care. But if someone's condition is the opposite, one should bleed him with caution and care. *De venae sectione.*[2]

بسم الله الرحمن الرحيم

رب يسّر

المقالة الثانية عشر

تشتمل على فصول تتعلّق

باستفراغ بإخراج الدم

٥

١. بهذه الثلاثة أشياء قوام الاستدلال على الحاجة إلى الفصد وهي عظم الأمراض الحاضرة أو المتوقّع حدوثها والسن وهولا يكون شيخا ولا صبيا وشدّة القوة. في مقالته في الفصد.

٢. من كانت عروقه من الناس واسعة غليظة وكان في بدنه بعض القضف ولم يكن لونه أبيض ولا كان له رطبا فينبغي أن يقدم على فصده بلا توقّ ولا حذر. ومن كانت حاله ضدّ هذه الحال فليستعمل الفصد فيه بتوقّ وحذر. في مقالته في الفصد.

١٠

---

١ بسم الله الرحمن الرحيم رب يسّر [.om ELBOU

(3) Do not bleed children below fourteen years, nor [anyone] older than seventy. Do not consider the number of years only, but also the external condition [of the body],[3] because some people are [only] sixty years old and yet cannot tolerate venesection, while others who are seventy can tolerate it, because they have much blood and their strength is great. But in spite of this, you should only extract a small amount of blood, even if their blood is like that of those who are in the prime of their life.[4] *De venae sectione.*[5]

(4) It is a general rule, for anyone [whom] one wants to bleed in the beginning of spring, that one examine and interrogate him. If he has a weak organ and his body is full [of superfluous matter], this fullness will tend to that weak organ. Then one should bleed him from the side opposite that weak organ in order to draw the [superfluous] matters away from it. But if he does not have such an organ, one may bleed him from whatever spot one likes. *De venae sectione.*[6]

(5) One should not proceed to perform venesection, even if there are clear signs of overfilling, under the following bodily conditions and symptoms: [someone suffering from] spasms, severe sleeplessness, heavy pain, severe heat, or severe cold; [those residing in] countries that are extremely hot or cold; [someone with] a very hot and dry temperament; someone whose flesh is lax, soft and flabby,[7] and dissolves quickly; someone who is extremely fat or extremely lean; someone who is young or old; someone who is faint-hearted; someone who is not used to bleeding; someone whose cardia of the stomach is so painful that he is weakened by indigestions and suffering from burning bad humors; or someone who has diarrhea. But when the body of a patient is very full [of blood] besides [having] one of these [bodily] conditions, bleeding him is unavoidable. But one should [only] bleed a small amount with caution and care. These questions are elucidated in *Ad Glauconem [de methodo medendi]* 1,[8] and all these [conditions] lead to weakness of the animal faculty.[9]

٣. لا تقصد الصبي قبل أربعة عشر سنة ولا بعد السبعين ولا تنظر إلى عدد السنين فقط بل انظر مع ذلك في السحنة، فإنك تجد قوما لهم الستين سنة لا يحتملون الفصد وتجد قوما لهم سبعون سنة يحتملونه لأنك تجدهم دمهم كثيرا وقوتهم قوية ومع ذلك فلا تستفرغ من دمهم إلا قليل وإن كان دمهم كدم المتناهين. في مقالته في الفصد.

٤. أمر عام لجميع من يقصد فصده في ابتداء الربيع وهو أن يتأمّل الشخص الذي يفصده ويسأله. فمتى كان بعض أعضائه ضعيفا من شأنه متى امتلأ بدنه أن يميل الامتلاء نحو ذلك العضو الضعيف. فافصد من الجهة التي تقابل ذلك العضو الضعيف لتجذب المواد عنه. ومتى لم يكن بعض أعضائه كذلك فافصده من أيّ مواضع أحبّ. في مقالته في الفصد.

٥. الأحوال والأعراض التي لا تقدم معها على إخراج الدم وإن كانت علامات الامتلاء ظاهرة هي هذه: تشنّج أو الأرق الشديد أو الوجع المؤلم أو الحرّ الشديد أو البرد الشديد أو البلدان الحارّة جدًا أو الباردة جدًا أو المزاج الحارّ اليابس جدًا أو من كان له لينا رخوا سخيفا سريع التحلّل أو من أفرط عليه السمن أو من أفرط عليه الهزال أو من كان صبيا أو شيخا أو من كان خوّارا أو من لم تجد عادة بإخراج الدم أو من فم معدته متألّما أنهكته التخم أو تلذعه أخلاط رديئة أو من معه ذرب. ومتى كان العليل ممتلئا جدًا مع حالة من هذه الحالات ولم يكن بدّ من الفصد فاخرج له بحذر وتوقّ شيئا قليلا. تلخّصت هذه المسائل في الأولى من أغلوقن وهي كلّها تؤول إلى ضعف القوة الحيوانية.

---

٣ ومع...المتناهين] U¹ : ELO .om ‖ ٦ امتلأ] بدأ L ‖ ٨ الضعيف] G¹ ‖ ١٦ حالة] واحدة L ‖ ١٧ المسائل] الشرائط ELBOU

(6) When the body is full of raw humors, it is very dangerous to apply venesection, because the strength [of the patient] is so greatly weakened and undermined that it is absolutely impossible for his body to return to its previous condition—and especially so if the patient also has fever. *De venae sectione.*[10]

(7) If someone's body contains a small amount of good blood and a very large quantity of raw humors, [venesection should not be applied],[11] and he should not carry out any activity at all and not enter the bathhouse. For venesection removes the good blood from [the body] and attracts the bad blood collected in the primary [nonpulsatile] vessels of the liver and disperses it throughout the body. When one gives a purgative to such a patient, it causes colic, biting pain, and fainting, but it does not evacuate anything in a [significant] quantity.[12] For the humors precede [the matter to be evacuated] and obstruct the passages because of their thickness. For this reason, he should not exercise nor enter the bathhouse. But the humors of such patients should be thinned and cut with ingredients that do not heat excessively. *De sanitate tuenda* 4.[13]

(8) When a person is healthy but has signs of overfilling, it does not necessarily mean that we have to bleed him. Rather, for such a person, one should limit oneself and be content with withholding food [from him].[14] In the case of someone else, one should limit oneself to diminishing his food [intake], and in yet another, one should limit oneself to prescribing laxatives or purgatives, or frequent bathing in the bathhouse, or exercise only, or much massage—each person according to his fullness[15] and habit. One should be content to apply one of these so that one need not apply bleeding. *De methodo [medendi]* 4.[16]

(9) Regarding venesection, one should know that in the case of someone who has little blood, one should first of all treat him by improving his humors. Then one can apply venesection to him and feed him subsequently. If necessary, one may bleed him again. This therapy is most appropriate for someone whose blood is turbid or contains a thick sediment. *De methodo [medendi]* 5.[17]

٦. إذا كان البدن مملوًءا أخلاطٍ نيئة فالخطر في الفصد عظيمًا فإنّ القوة تضعف وتسترخي في الغاية القصوى حتّى لا يمكن أصلًا أن يرجع البدن إلى حالتها الأولى وخاصّة متى كان مع ذلك حمّى. في مقالته في الفصد.

٧. البدن الذي يكون الدم الجيّد فيه قليلًا والأخلاط النيئة كثيرة جدًّا لا ينبغي أن يتحرّك بشيء أصلًا ولا يدخل حمّامًا. وذلك أنّ الفصد يخرج الدم الجيّد منه ويجذب الدم الرديء المجتمع في العروق الأوّل التي في الكبد ويبثه في البدن كلّه. فأمّا الدواء المسهل فيحدث لصاحب هذه الحال مغصًا ولذعًا وغشيًا ولا يستفرغ شيئًا له قدر. والأخلاط لغلظها تسبق وتسدّ المجاري ولهذا السبب لا ينبغي أن يرتاض ولا يدخل حمّامًا. وإنّما ينبغي أن ترقّق أخلاطهم وتقطع بما لا يسخن إسخانًا كثيرًا. رابعة تدبير الصحّة.

٨. الإنسان إذا كان صحيحًا وكانت دلائل الامتلاء موجودة فليس يضطرّنا الأمر لإخراج الدم ولا بدّ. بل تقتصر في ذلك الشخص على الإمساك عن الطعام فكتفي بذلك. واقصر في آخره على تقليل الطعام واقتصر بآخره على إلانة البطن أو على الإسهال أو على الإكثار من الحمّام أو على الرياضة وحدها أو على الدلك الكثير، كلّ شخص بحسب امتلائه وعادته. ويكتفي بذلك عن إخراج الدم. رابعة الحيلة.

٩. أمّا الفصد فينبغي لك أن تعرف من أمره أنّ من كان قليل الدم فينبغي لك أن تداويه أوّلًا بأن تجوّد أخلاطه. ثمّ يمكنك بعد ذلك أن تقصده العرق وتغذوه بعد الفصد، ثمّ تقصده أيضًا إن احتاج لذلك. وأولى الناس أن يفعل به هذا من كان في دمه عكرًا أو ثفل راسب غليظ. خامسة الحيلة.

١ الفصد] ذلك G || ٤ النيّة] فيه add. ELO || ٥ يتحرّك] يحرك ELBOU الجيّد منه ويجذب الدم] G¹ || ١٢ ذلك الشخص] شخص G ذلك : B عن] على G || ١٣ واقصر] ويقتصر ELO || ١٥ امتلائه] احتماله ELU || ١٦ لك] om. ELO قليل] رديء ELBO بأن] حتّى L

(10) If, during a venesection, it happens to a person that the mouth of a [nonpulsatile] vessel bursts open, or that menstruation sets in, or that diarrhea develops, one should consider its quantity and vehemence. For, if this is sufficient for the amount needed to be evacuated, let nature take care of the complete evacuation. But if you see that it is less than what needs to be evacuated, you should empty [again] through venesection such a quantity as makes both evacuations together enough to get the required amount. *De methodo [medendi]* 9.[18]

(11) If bleeding is required but indigestion occurs, one should postpone the bleeding until the food is digested and its superfluities are excreted from the body. If another [type of] evacuation occurs, it is absolutely necessary to postpone [the bleeding]. *De methodo [medendi]* 9.[19]

(12) If the chymes have increased evenly, evacuate all of them equally. The most proper way to do so is, above all, through venesection, closely followed by the evacuation effected through scarification of the ankle.[20] Next comes that effected through exercise, massage, bathing in the bathhouse, and abstention from food. *In Hippocratis Aphorismos commentarius* 2.[21]

(13) When you know that the body contains a surplus of seething blood, you should evacuate it quickly before it streams to one of the major[22] organs. Therefore, you should not refrain from applying venesection when necessary, whether it is day or night. *De venae sectione.*[23]

(14) It often happens that blood, before it putrefies, suddenly streams to one of the organs because of its surplus and either mortifies it completely, so that its function is annulled, or causes it severe damage, such as [occurs in] the disease of apoplexy. For this disease originates from a large quantity of blood streaming to the brain. Therefore, when signs of a surplus of blood become evident, along with strength of the faculties— that is, the psychical, animal,[24] and natural ones—carry out venesection without any caution. *De venae sectione.*[25]

١٠. إن اتفق أن يحدث لشخص انفتاح أفواه العروق أو يدرّ الطمث أو يلين الطبع في وقت استعمال الفصد فانظر كيّة ذلك أو اندفاعه. فإن كان يفي باستفراغ ما يجب استفراغه فدع الطبيعة تتولّى الاستفراغ كلّه. وإن رأيت أن ذلك أقلّ ممّا يحتاج فاستفرغه أنت بالفصد بمقدار ما يفي إلا استفراغان جميعا بمقدار الحاجة. تاسعة الحيلة.

١١. إذا وجب الفصد وحدثت تخمة فينبغي أن يؤخّر أمر الفصد إلى أن يستمرأ ذلك الطعام وتخرج فضلته عن البدن. فإن كان حدث استفراغ آخر لزم التأخير باضطرار. تاسعة الحيلة.

١٢. إذا كانت الكيموسات قد تزيّدت على التناسب فاستفرغ كلّها بالسوى. وأصحّ ما يكون ذلك بالفصد خاصّة ويقرب منه الذي يكون بالشرط على الكاحل وبعده الذي يكون بالرياضة والدلك والحمّام وترك الطعام. في شرحه لثانية الفصول.

١٣. يجب عليك متى علمت أنّ في البدن كثرة من الدم قد غلى أن تسرع استفراغه قبل أن ينصبّ إلى بعض الأعضاء النفيسة. ولذلك لا ينبغي لك أن تمنع من فصد العرق متى احتجت إلى ذلك ليلا كان أو نهارا. في مقالته في الفصد.

١٤. كثيرا ما ينصبّ الدم لكثرته بغتة قبل أن يعفن لعضو من الأعضاء فيميته أصلا فيبطل فعله أو يحدث عليه ضررا عظيما مثل علّة السكتة. فإنّ حدوثها يكون عن انصباب دم كثير إلى الدماغ بغتة. فإذا ظهرت أمارات كثرة الدم مع قوة هذه الثلاث قوى يعني النفسانية والحيوانية والطبيعية فتقدم على الفصد من غير حذر. في مقالته في الفصد.

١ إن...في مقالته في الفصد (١٣) E .om || ٢ كيّة : G جهد | BU حمية | يفي | يفيد B || ٦ حدث L .om || ٧ تاسعة الحيلة] في تلك المقالة L || ٩ الكاحل] Bos .emend : الكاهل MSS: כאהל N || ١٠ وترك] وبترك LBOU || ١١ يجب عليك] ينبغي لك L ينبغي عليك O || ١٢ النفيسة] النقية B || ١٥ علّة] علل G || ١٦ عن] عند ELBOU

(15) When the body contains a large quantity of blood that has become extremely hot and seething and causes acute fever, one should evacuate a large quantity of blood at one stroke to the point of syncope, after examining the greatness of the strength [of the patient]. I know that I have personally evacuated about five *raṭls* [immediately or] on the second, third, or fourth day since the beginning of the fever.[26] *De venae sectione.*[27]

(16) If someone whose strength is weak needs the evacuation of a large quantity of blood, the best thing is to do so in many sessions, either in a single day or on a second and third day [as well]. Feed him after every evacuation with fine food. Be careful not to evacuate a large quantity at one time unless you are forced to do so for a very strong reason. *De venae sectione.*[28]

(17) If you want to simply evacuate blood, do so on the day of the bleeding.[29] But if you want to draw someone's blood in a contrary direction,[30] it is better to repeat it [i.e., to do so] on the second and third day.[31] In all [such] cases, you should consider the strength of the patient. *De venae sectione.*[32]

(18) If you perform a venesection and the blood is streaming, pay attention to a change in its color, especially if [the patient] suffers from an inflamed tumor. You should also pay attention to a reduction in the intensity of the flow[33] of the blood. But above all, pay attention to a change[34] of the pulse. If you see that it changes in either volume or regularity, stop the bleeding. But a change toward weakness is something I do not have to discuss.[35] *De venae sectione.*[36]

(19) In all diseases, you should, once you have evacuated a moderate amount of blood, attempt to repeat this either on the first day (when possible) or on the second day, unless you intend to evacuate to the point of syncope. *De venae sectione.*[37]

١٥. متى كان في البدن من الدم مقدار كثير قد اشتدّت سخونته وغلى فأحدث حتى حاذة فاستفرغ دماً كثيرا دفعة إلى أن يعرض الغشي بعد أن تتفقد شدّة القوة. وإني لأعرف أني استفرغت في اليوم الثاني من ابتداء الحمى نحو خمسة أرطال أو في اليوم الثالث أو في اليوم الرابع. في مقالته في الفصد.

١٦. الأصلح لمن يحتاج أن يستفرغ منه دم كثير والقوة منه ضعيفة أن يستفرغ في دفعات كثيرة إمّا في يوم واحد أو في الثاني والثالث وتغذوه بعد كلّ استفراغ بغذاء لطيف. وينبغي لك أن تحذر الاستفراغ الكثير دفعة متى لم يضطرك لذلك أمر عظيم. في مقالته في الفصد.

١٧. إن كان قصدك استفراغ الدم مطلقا فاجعله في يوم الفصد. فأمّا من تقصد فيه الجذب إلى خلاف الجهة فإن التثنية في اليوم الثاني والثالث أجود. وتفقد في كلّ حال قوة المريض. في مقالته في الفصد.

١٨. إذا فصدت العرق وجرى الدم فتفقد تغيّر لونه وبخاصّة إذا كان بالإنسان ورم حارّ. وتفقد أيضا حمية خروج الدم إذا انقطعت، وأكثر من جميع ذلك تفقد حال النبض. فإذا رأيت النبض قد تغيّر إمّا في عظمه وإمّا في استوائه فاقطع إخراج الدم. وأمّا تغيّره إلى الضعف فليس لي حاجة إلى ذكره. في مقالته في الفصد.

١٩. ينبغي أن تروم في جميع العلل بعد أن تستفرغ من الدم مقدارا معتدلا أن تستعمل التثنية إمّا في اليوم الأوّل إذا أمكن ذلك وإمّا في اليوم الثاني اللهمّ إلا أن تقصد الاستفراغ إلى أن يبلغ الغشي. في مقالته في الفصد.

١ متى] إذا L: إن O: إن ... متى] متى ... في مقالته في الفصد E .om || ٤ في اليوم] L .om || ٦ أو في الثاني والثالث] أو في الثلاث L || ٩ الفصد] القصد B || ١٠ التثنية] التثنه B(!): G(؟)

(20) When someone is trained and experienced in the medical practice, he should not refrain from bloodletting when the illness is severe
and serious and the patient has great strength. [He should do so] even
if there are no signs of overfilling, but only a severe and serious disease.
The same applies to the application of purgatives or emetics, either
because of a surplus of humors other than blood or because of the severity
and seriousness of the illness, in order to draw this surplus to the opposite side [and to evacuate it] and to support the strength [of the patient].
De methodo [medendi] 4.[38]

(21) Bloodletting always needs great strength, equivalent to the
amount to be evacuated. [Lack of] strength is the most dangerous of
all things [in the case of bloodletting]. When, in the case of continuous
fever resulting from the impossibility of dissolution,[39] one's strength is
great, bloodletting is mostly safe, far from being dangerous. But in
other illnesses, bloodletting is dangerous, and a patient may suffer from
very severe afflictions because of it. *De methodo [medendi]* 9.[40]

(22) You were often in my presence when I ordered bleeding someone who suffered from either podagra or arthritis or epilepsy or melancholy or chronic hemoptysis; or someone whose chest condition was
such that he would easily fall victim to such a disease; or someone suffering from obstruction, or frequent angina, or inflammation of the
lungs, or pleurisy, or inflammation of the liver, or severe ophthalmia.
For venesection is necessary in all these illnesses at their onset. Similarly, in the case of anyone losing blood from the mouths of his vessels
and then stopping, bleed him with confidence and trust. Similarly, in
the case of a woman whose menstruation stops or of someone who suffers from a nosebleed, hasten to bleed such persons, [taking into] con-
sideration their strength and age. *De venae sectione.*[41]

(23) When someone suffers from ulcerous fatigue,[42] blood should be
evacuated to the point of fainting, if there is no contraindication. One[43]
should examine [the patient]; and when he finds that the patient feels
tension and pricking pain in his chest, back, and loins, he should bleed

٢٠. متى كان المرض شديدا صعبا وكانت القوة قوية لا يمتنع أحد ممّن راض نفسه واحتنك في أعمال الطبّ من إخراج الدم ولا يوقف عنه وإن لم تكن هناك دلائل تدلّ على الامتلاء لكن من أجل شدّة المرض وصعوبته فقط. وكذلك استعمل إسهال البطن والقيء إنّما بسبب كثرة أخلاط أخرى سوى الدم أو بسبب شدّة المرض وصعوبته لتجذب إلى خلاف الجهة أو لتخفّف عن القوة. رابعة الحيلة.

٢١. إخراج الدم أبدا يحتاج إلى قوة قوية تفي بمقدار الاستفراغ. والقوة أجلّ خطرا من جميع الأشياء والحمّى المطبقة التي تكون من قبل امتناع التحلّل لما كانت القوة فيها على أكثر الأمر مرقوقة صار الاستفراغ فيها مأمون العاقبة بعيدا عن المخاطرة. وأمّا في الأمراض الأخرى فالاستفراغ مخاطرة وصاحبه يقع منه إلى غاية البلاء. تاسعة الحيلة.

٢٢. قد حضرتموني كثيرا آمر بفصد من به النقرس أو وجع المفاصل أو الصرع أو المالنخوليا أو نفث الدم المتقادم أو من كانت هيئة صدره هيئة يسهل معها وقوعه في هذا المرض أو من به سدد أو من يعرض له الاختناق كثيرا أو ورم الرئة أو الشوصة أو ورم الكبد أو رمد شديد. فإنّ فصد العرق في جميع هذه العلل في أوّل حدوثها يضطرّ إليه. وكذلك كلّ من يأتيه دم من أفواه العروق وانقطع، اقدم على فصده بثقة وأمن. وكذلك المرأة التي انقطع طمثها أو من به رعاف بادر بفصده مع النظر في القوة والسنّ. في مقالته في الفصد.

٢٣. صاحب الإعياء الورمي ينبغي أن يستفرغ الدم حتّى يبلغ الغشي إن لم يمنع من ذلك مانع. وينظر إن وجد التمدّد والنخس يحسّ بهما في الصدر والصلب

---

١ متى] ما .add ELO || ٦ أبدا] أبتداء EL || ٧ المطبقة] المحرقة ELBU || ١٠ كثيرا] مرارا L || ١١ المالنخوليا] المالنخونيا EL || ١٢ به] .om ELBO || من] .om ELO || ١٣ في] .om ELBOU

the basilic vein. But when the patient feels this in the head and neck, he should bleed the cephalic vein. And when [the patient] feels the fatigue equally throughout the body, he should bleed the median vein. *De sanitate tuenda* 4.[44]

(24) When a nerve tears in its width, the patient is in danger of [suffering from] spasms when an [inflamed] tumor develops. Therefore, one should remove blood from this patient without compassion and in a larger quantity than one would in the case of another illness. And one should prescribe him a regimen of the finest possible food and of rest. One should also apply plenty of hot olive oil, from the site of the wound to the roots of that nerve [and] on the spine[45] up to the neck. *De methodo [medendi]* 6.[46]

(25) If someone lets blood because of a fever, he should do so during the decline of the [fever] attack, day or night. Beware of letting blood while food is still present in the stomach and as long as the humors in the stomach and first [nonpulsatile] vessels are not [completely] cocted. But for someone who does not have fever, such as someone who has ophthalmia, the best time for letting blood is when the pain is severe. And if there is no pain, the best time is at daybreak, one hour after waking up. *De venae sectione.*[47]

(26) When bleeding someone suffering from a fever, do not consider the number of days that have passed since [the beginning of] the illness, whether it is the fourth or fifth day. Rather, when you find that the patient is fit for bleeding,[48] you should bleed him at that moment, even if it is the twentieth day since the beginning of the illness. You can find out about that [i.e., the patient's fitness] from the severity of the illness, the greatness of the strength [of the patient], the support of the age [of the patient], and the time [of the year]. *De venae sectione.*[49]

(27) When someone complains about an illness in the parts below the collarbone, it is most appropriate to bleed him from the basilic-axillary vein. And when someone complains about an illness in the parts above the collarbone, it is most appropriate to bleed him from the humeral vein. *De anatomia magna* 3.[50]

والقطن فيفصد الباسليق. وإن كان يحسّهما في الرأس والرقبة فينبغي أن يفصد القيفال. وإن كان حسّ الإعياء في البدن كلّه بالسوى فيفصد الأكحل. رابعة تدبير الصحّة.

٢٤. متى انخرقت العصبة في عرضها فإنّ صاحبها على خطر من التشنّج إذا حدث الورم. ولذلك ينبغي أن يخرج لصاحبها من الدم بلا رحمة أكثر ممّا يخرج لغيره ويدبّر بألطف ما يمكن من الغذاء ويلزم الهدوء والتغريق بالدهن المسخن من موضع الجراحة إلى أصول تلك العصبة إلى الظهر إلى الرقبة. سادسة الحيلة.

٢٥. من يفصد من أجل الحمّى فينبغي أن يفصد في وقت انحطاط النوبة ليلاً كان أو نهارا. وإيّاك والفصد والطعام في المعدة حتّى تنضج الأخلاط التي في المعدة وفي العرق الأوّل التي قد نضجت بعض نضج. وأمّا من لا حمّى به كالأرمد فأجود الأوقات لفصده وقت شدّة الوجع. وإن لم يكن ثمّ وجع فأجود الأوقات أوائل النهار بعد الانتباه بساعة. في مقالته في الفصد.

٢٦. لا تنظر في فصد المحموم الذي ينبغي فصده في عدد الأيّام الماضية من المرض لا رابع ولا خامس. بل متى وجدت أنّ المريض أهلاً للفصد افصده في ذلك الوقت وإن كان اليوم العشرين مثلاً منذ ابتداء المرض. وتعلم ذلك بعظم المرض وشدّة القوة ومساعدة السن والزمان. في مقالته في الفصد.

٢٧. أصلح ما يفصد لمن يشكو علّة في الأعضاء التي أسفل من الترقوة الباسليق الإبطي. وأصلح ما يفصد لمن يشكو علّة في الأعضاء التي فوق الترقوة العرق الكتفي. في ثلاثة التشريح الكبير.

---

٧ سادسة] سابعة L || ١٠ العرق] العروق ELBOU | كالأرمد] كالرمد L : كالماد E : كالأزمة B || ١٨ الترقوة] التراقي G

(28) For illnesses in the parts above the liver, bleeding should be done [from the vein] at the inner side of the arm; and for illnesses of the parts below the liver, [from the vein] at the inner side of the knee or from the saphenous vein. *In Hippocratis Epidemiarum* 6.1.[51]

5   (29) For an [inflamed] tumor in the side [of the body], lungs, diaphragm, spleen, liver, or stomach, one derives clear benefit by bloodletting from the basilic vein. For the lower parts, such as those which lie next to the hip, the urinary bladder, and uterus, one should bleed [from the vein] at the inner side of the knee[52] or at the ankle. Since the kid-

10   neys lie in the middle between these parts, one is benefitted by bleeding [from the vein] at the inner side of the arm,[53] [provided] this is done when the inflammation is recent and when the whole body is filled with blood. But when the [inflamed] tumor in the kidneys becomes prolonged and old, one should bleed from the vein in the inner side of the

15   knee or alongside the ankle. *De venae sectione.*[54]

(30) When ischias is caused by a surplus of blood, do not start with any kind of treatment before evacuating the surplus. Do not be content with evacuating the blood from the leg only, but also [do so] from the inner side of the elbow. *Mayāmir* 10.[55]

20   (31) As for bloodletting from the saphenous vein or from the one at the inner side of the knee,[56] I know that the illness called sciatica is cured in one day through the evacuation of blood from the leg, when it is caused by overfilling with blood. But cupping is of no benefit to such patients.[57] *De venae sectione.*[58]

25   (32) When you want to stop the bleeding from the mouths of the vessels, you should let blood from the veins in the arms. If you want to stimulate it, you should bleed from the veins in the legs. Similarly, you should always bleed from these veins[59] to induce menstruation. When vessels in the uterus burst (because of an erosion or because of overfill-

30   ing) and the woman loses blood and you want to stop the bleeding, you should let blood from the veins in the arms, since this is not menstrual blood [which we would like to stimulate]. *De venae sectione.*[60]

٢٨. الفصد ينبغي أن يستعمل في علل الأعضاء التي فوق الكبد من مأبض اليد وفي علل الأعضاء التي تحت الكبد من مأبض الركبة ومن الصافن. في الأولى من شرحه لسادسة أبيديميا.

٢٩. ورم الجنب أو الرئة أو الحجاب أو الطحال أو الكبد أو المعدة فالمنفعة تكون فيها بيّنة بفصد الباسليق. والأعضاء السفلية منها كالأعضاء التي تلي الورك والمثانة والرحم فيفصد فيها من باطن الركبة ومن فوق الكعب. وأمّا الكلى فإنها واسطة بين هذه الأعضاء فلذلك قد ينتفع فيها بالفصد من مأبض اليد بقرب عهد حدوث الورم فيها وإن كان جميع البدن مملوءا دما. فأمّا إذا طال وقدم الورم في الكلى فافصد العرق التي في باطن الركبة أو على الكعب. في مقالته في الفصد.

٣٠. إذا كان سبب عرق النساء كثرة الدم فلا تبتدئ بشيء قبل استفراغه ولا تقتصر على استفراغ الدم من الرجل دون أن تستفرغه أيضا من باطن المرفق. عاشرة الميامر.

٣١. أمّا فصد العرق الصافن أو الذي في باطن الركبة فإني لا أعلم أنّ العلة التي تسمّى عرق النساء برئت في يوم واحد عند استفراغ الدم من الرجل وذلك إذا كان سببها امتلاء من الدم. وأمّا الحجامة هناك فلا تنفعهم. في مقالته في الفصد.

٣٢. الدم الذي يجري من أفواه العروق إن أردت قطعه فافصد العروق التي في اليدين وإن أردت إدراره فافصد العروق التي في الرجلين. وكذلك تقصدها دائما لإدرار الطمث. وأمّا إن انبثقت عروق في الرحم من تأكّل أو من امتلاء ونزفت المرأة دما وأردت قطع ذلك الدم فافصد العروق التي في اليدين إذ وليس ذلك دم طمث. في مقالته في الفصد.

---

٣ أبيديميا] أفيديميا ELOU ‖ ١٣ لأعلم] لا أعلم G ‖ ٢٠ في الفصد] تلك EL

(33) When an [inflamed] tumor begins in the liver, chest, or lungs, bleed from the basilic vein in the right arm. If this vein is not clearly visible, do so from the median vein; and if this one is not clearly visible, do so from the cephalic vein. When an [inflamed] tumor starts to develop in the parts of the mouth,[61] bleed from the cephalic vein. If this one is not clearly visible, do so from the median vein; and if this one is not clearly visible, from the basilic vein. In the case of angina, as a last resort, let blood from [the jugular vein] under the tongue. *De methodo [medendi]* 13.[62]

(34) When the illness is in the nape of the neck,[63] let blood from the arm or from the forehead. In the case of [inflamed] tumors in the kidneys or uterus, let blood from the vein that is at the inner side of the knee. If this is not possible, then [bleed] from the vein alongside the ankle— namely, the saphenous.[64] For illnesses of the spleen, let blood from the left arm. *De methodo [medendi]* 13.[65]

(35) When the spleen is affected, bloodletting from the vein between the little finger and ring finger of the left hand is of great benefit. The same holds good for bloodletting from the basilic vein[66] of the left arm. However, do not evacuate the amount that you wish to remove at one time, but over two days. *De venae sectione.*[67]

(36) When, in the case of someone suffering from pleurisy, one bleeds from a vein on the same side as[68] the inflammation, it sometimes[69] brings clear benefit. But when one lets blood from the arm opposite to the ill- ness, the benefit is not noticeable or only becomes visible after a long time. The same applies to severe pain in the eyes, for bloodletting from the cephalic vein on the same side alleviates the pain immediately and is of great benefit. *De venae sectione.*[70]

(37) When you bleed someone suffering from a nosebleed or apply cupping glasses to his forehead and the nosebleed did not stop, you should not hastily cool his head; rather, put cupping glasses on the occipital protuberance on the back of his head, because it attracts [the blood] to the opposite side. *De methodo [medendi]* 5.[71]

(38) For chronic illnesses of the head or eyes that are caused by hot, fine matter, one sometimes lets blood from the pulsatile vessels in the temples or behind the ears, especially when these illnesses occur

٣٣. في ابتداء ورم الكبد والصدر والرئة افصد الباسليق من اليد اليمنى وإن لم يتبيَّن فالأَكحل وإن لم يتبيَّن فالقيفال. وإن ابتدأ الورم في أعضاء الفم فافصد القيفال وإن لم يتبيَّن فالأَكحل وإن لم يتبيَّن فالباسليق وآخر الأمر يفصد في الخوانيق تحت اللسان. ثالثة عشر الحيلة.

٣٤. متى كانت العلة في القفاء فافصد من اليد أو من الجبهة. وفي أورام الكليتين والأرحام تقصد العرق الذي في مأبض الركبة. فإن لم يتهيأ فالعرق الذي في الكعب وهو الصافن. وفي علل الطحال تقصد من اليد اليسرى. ثالثة عشر الحيلة.

٣٥. إذا اعتلَّ الطحال ففصد العرق الذي بين الخنصر والبنصر من اليد اليسرى نافع جدًا وكذلك فصد الباسليق من اليد اليسرى. ولا تستفرغ ما تريد استفراغه دفعة بل في يومين. في مقالته في الفصد.

٦٣. فصد العرق في من به الشوصة إذا كان محاذيًا للجانب الذي الورم فيه فقد تظهر منفعة كثيرة. وإذا كان من اليد المقابلة للعلّة فالانتفاع به يكون خفيا أو يكون ظهوره بعد زمان طويل. وكذلك أوجاع العين الشديدة أيضا فإنَّ فصد القيفال الحاذّي لها يسكّنه في ساعته وينتفع به منفعة عظيمة. في مقالته في الفصد.

٣٧. إن كنت فصدت لصاحب الرعاف أو علّقت على جبهته المحاجم فلم ينقطع الرعاف فلا تبادر بتبريد الرأس بل تعلّق مجّة في موضع الفأس من مؤخّر الدماغ فإنّه يجذب إلى خلاف الجهة. خامسة الحيلة.

٣٨. العروق الضوارب التي في الصدغين وخلف الأذنين قد تقصد في علل الرأس أو العينين المزمنة إذا كان سبب العلل مادّة حارّة لطيفة وبخاصّة إذا كان

٢ فالأَكحل وإن لم يتبيَّن] G¹ [الفم] العليا B || ٥ في] من L || ٩ نافع جدًا]
om. G [وكذلك فصد الباسليق من اليد اليسرى] om. B : وكذلك الباسليق من اليد اليسرى
G¹ || ١٤ في] من ELO || ١٦ الفأس] الرأس ELB

in the membranes.[72] In these illnesses, the patient feels as if he is being
pricked, and then this pain spreads out, while the pricking sensation
remains in the center of that site. However, bloodletting from pulsatile
vessels is very dangerous because sometimes the [flow of] blood does not
5   stop or an aneurysm[73] develops. For this reason, physicians avoid bleeding from a large pulsatile vessel (and also from a small one) because it is
of little benefit. When a pulsatile vessel is cut widthwise, it is not dangerous because every part contracts to its own side. *De venae sectione.*[74]

       (39) If a surplus of thick blood, or blood with another reprehensible
10 quality, collects in the [nonpulsatile] vessels, you should first of all apply
venesection and then, as a second thing, use a purgative that cleanses the
[thick] humor[ous part] within the blood. *In Hippocratis Epidemiarum 6.1.*[75]

       (40) When, in the case of melancholic delusion and the like, all the
indications suggest to you that the blood in all the [nonpulsatile] vessels
15 is melancholic, you should bleed from the median cubital vein. If the
blood [that flows out] is not melancholic, stop bleeding immediately.
If you observe it to be melancholic, withdraw as much as you think the
body of the patient can tolerate. This is a most important diagnostic
rule.[76] *De locis affectis 3.*[77]

20   (41) You should not first administer any strong remedy to patients
with quartan fevers, nor desire to evacuate their bodies, unless you
observe a surplus of blood that strongly prevails. When you let blood,
examine it, and if you see that it is black and thick, evacuate with assur-
ance and assiduity. But if you see that it is pure red[78] and thin, stop its
25 extraction. *Ad Glauconem [de methodo medendi] 1.*[79]

حدوثها في الأغشية التي يحسّ الإنسان كأنّه يخس ثمّ ينبسط ذلك الوجع ويبق النفس في مركز ذلك الموضع. لكن أخطار فصد العروق الضوارب عظيمة لأنّه قد لا ينقطع الدم أو يحدث أمّ الدم. ولهذا السبب هرب الأطباء من فصد ما كان منها عظيما ومن فصد ما كان منها صغيرا لأنّ منفعته يسيرة. وإذا بتر العرق الضارب في عرضه فلا خطر فيه لأنّه يتقلّص كل واحد من طرفيه إلى الجانب الذي هو فيه. في

٥

مقالته في الفصد.

٣٩. إذا اجتمع دم كثير غليظ أو له كيفية أخرى مذمومة في العروق فينبغي أن تبتدئ بالفصد، ثمّ تثني باستعمال الدواء المسهل المنقّي للخلط الذي في الدم. في الأولى من شرحه لسادسة أبيديميا.

٤٠. إذا دلّتك الدلائل العامّة في الوسواس السوداوي ونحوه أنّ الدم الذي في العروق كلّها صار سوداويا فافصد الأكحل. فإن كان الدم الذي يجري ليس

١٠

بسوداوي فاقطعه وامنعه على المكان. وإن رأيته سوداويا فأخرج منه بمقدار ما يظنّ أن بدن العليل يكتفي به. وهذا الباب أبلغ ما يكون في التعرّف. ثالثة التعرّف.

٤١. أصحاب الربع في أول الأمر لا تسقيهم شيئا من الأدوية القوية ولا تروم استفراغ أبدانهم اللهمّ إلّا أن ترى الدم كثيرا غالبا جدّا. وإذا فصدت تفقد الدم

١٥

وإن رأيته أسود غليظا فثق وتقدّم على الإمعان في الاستفراغ. وإن رأيته ناصع الحمرة رفيقا فاقطع إخراجه. أولى أغلوقن.

٢ مركز] مؤخّر L || ٣ أمّ] om. B || ٨ في] فيه L | الدم] الورم E || ٩ أبيديميا] أفيديميا ELOU || ١٢ بمقدار] G¹ || ١٣ العليل] المريض ELBOU

(42) In the case of women who develop dropsy because of the retention of their menstruation, as well as in the case of those in whom dropsy occurs because of a retention of the blood that was streaming from the mouths of the veins or through a nosebleed, one should hurry to bleed them before their strength dissolves and collapses. *In Hippocratis Epidemiarum* 6.7.[80]

(43) Sometimes, apply cupping glasses to the hollow in the back of the neck[81] to attract the matter which streams to the eyes [in the opposite direction][82] and bleed from the frontal vein to attract the matter which is in the posterior part of the head. *In Hippocratis De humoribus commentarius* 1.[83]

(44) If someone has a surplus of thick, melancholic blood, it is most appropriate, first of all, to bleed him and then to purge the black bile. When crude humors prevail in someone's body, evacuate his body with care and caution before the illness begins. But if he suffers from fever, do not evacuate at all. *De venae sectione.*[84]

(45) When you treat hardness of the spleen and the illness remains unchanged, apply cupping glasses after scarifying the site. Especially beneficial for hardness of the liver and spleen is to bleed from the vein above the left ear and then take from the extracted blood and rub it on the diseased spleen. *Mayāmir* 9.[85]

(46) When the chest, the brain, or the membranes of the brain suffer from an [inflamed] tumor, we do not apply cupping glasses in the beginning of the illness until we have stopped [superfluous] matter from arriving [at these sites] and have evacuated the entire body. For, then, the application of cupping glasses is very beneficial. But when the body is full, the cupping glasses attract the superfluous matter from the entire body and move it to the brain or the chest or the lungs, depending on where one has applied them. *De methodo [medendi]* 10.[86]

٤٢. النساء اللاتي يبتدئ بهنّ الاستسقاء بسبب احتباس الطمث وكذلك من عرض له ذلك من احتباس دم كان يجري من أفواه العروق أو رعاف ينبغي أن تبادر بفصدهم قبل أن تخلّ القوة وتسقط. في السابعة لشرحه لسادسة أبيذيميا.

٤٣. قد تعلّق المجمة على النقرة فتجذب المادّة التي تجري إلى العينين. وتقصد عرق الجبهة فتجذب المادّة التي تكون في مؤخّر الرأس. في الأولى من الأخلاط.

٤٤. من كان دمه غليظا سوداويا وكثيرا فالأولى أن تقصده أوّلا ثمّ تسهل السوداء. ومن كان الغالب في بدنه الأخلاط النيئة فاستفرغه قبل أن يحدث به المرض بتوقّ وحذر. وإذا حدثت به الحمّى فلا تقرب الاستفراغ أصلا. في مقالته في الفصد.

٤٥. متى داويت صلابة الطحال وبقيت العلّة على حالها فعلّق مجمة بعد أن تشرط الموضع وممّا ينفع صلابة الكبد والطحال بخاصّية أن يفصد العرق الذي من فوق الأذن اليسرى وتأخذ من الدم الذي يخرج وتدلك به الطحال العليل. تاسعة الميامر.

٤٦. متى حدث ورم في الصدر أو الدماغ أو أغشيته فإنّا لا نستعمل المحاجم في ابتداء العلّة لكن بعد أن نقطع مجيء المادّة ونستفرغ البدن كلّه وحينئذ تعليق المجمة نافع جدًا. وأمّا إن كان البدن ممتلئا جذبت المجمة الفضل من البدن كلّه وتورده على الدماغ أو الصدر أو الرئة حيث علّقت. حادية عشر الحيلة.

٣ أبيذيميا] أفيديميا ELOU ‖ ٦ وكثيرا] وكثّر ELU: عكر O

(47) If stretching [pain] is caused by a surplus of blood, such as occurs in the case of inflamed organs, one should bleed such a patient immediately. But if he is afraid of bloodletting or his strength is weak, one should draw the blood to the region opposite to that of the pain
5   through diversion.[87] *De methodo [medendi]* 12.[88]

This is the end of the twelfth treatise,
by the grace of God, praise be to Him.

◆

٤٧. متى كان السبب الفاعل للتمدد كثرة الدم بمنزلة ما يعرض ذلك للأعضاء الوارمة فينبغي أن يفصد لصاحبه عرق من ساعته. فإن جزع المريض من الفصد أو كانت قوته ضعيفة فيجذب الدم إلى الناحية المخالفة لناحية الوجع بالاستفراغ الناقل. ثانية عشر الحيلة.

تمت المقالة الثانية عشر ولله الحمد والمنة.

٥

---

٥ تمت المقالة الثانية عشر ولله الحمد والمنة] تمت المقالة الثانية عشر والحمد للة كثيرا E: كملت المقالة وعدد فصولها سبعة وأربعون فصلا L: تمت المقالة الثانية عشر B: تمت المقالة الرابعة عدد فصولها سبعة وأربعين U: كملت المقالة التاسعة عشر وعدد فصوها ألف الحمد لله على حسن ع ⟨...⟩ والسلام على المألفين من الله ⟨...⟩ تمّ الكتاب في سنت الف ט״ל לחרבן ב״ש תم ⟨...⟩ O

In the name of God,
the Merciful, the Compassionate.
O Lord, make [our task] easy

The Thirteenth Treatise

5   *Containing aphorisms concerning evacuations*
by means of purgatives and enemas

(1) All purgatives are harmful for the stomach and especially for the cardia, since it is very sensitive. Therefore, it is proper to mix purgatives with some fragrant substances. *In Hippocratis De acutorum morborum*
10   *[victu] et Galeni commentarius* 2.[1]

(2) Compound purgatives are bad[2] when one of the ingredients has a purgative effect as soon as the purgative enters the body, while another ingredient has this effect only long after its ingestion. *In Hippocratis De acutorum morborum [victu] et Galeni commentarius* 2.[3]

15   (3) Says Moses: Latex plants[4] and scammony [*Convolvulus scammonia*] purge as soon as they arrive in the body, whereas purgative resins purge only after a [prolonged] period. These resins are opopanax [gum resin of *Opopanax chironium* Koch], galbanum [gum resin of *Ferula galbaniflua*], sagapenum [gum resin of *Ferula scowitziana* and var.], asafetida [gum
20   resin of *Ferula asafoetida*], and gum ammoniacum [gum resin of *Ferula communis* var. *gummifera* or *F. tingitana*].

ربِّ يسِّر

المقالة الثالثة عشر

تشتمل على فصول تتعلَّق

بالاستفراغات بالأدوية المسهلة والحقن

٥

١. جميع الأدوية المسهلة تضرّ بالمعدة وبخاصة بفمها إذ كان أكثر حسًا.
ولذلك ينبغي أن يخلط بالأدوية المسهلة بعض الأدوية العطرة. في شرحه لثانية
الأمراض الحادة.

٢. فساد تركيب الأدوية المسهلة متى كان أحدها يسهل ساعة وروده البدن
والآخر بعد مدّة طويلة من تناوله. في شرحه لثانية الأمراض الحادة.

١٠

٣. قال موسى: إنَّ اليتوعات والمحمودة تسهل عند ورودها والصموغ المسهلة
تسهل بعد مدّة وهي الجاوشير والقنة والسكبينج والحلتيت والوشّق.

---

١ بسم الله الرحمن الرحيم ربِّ يسِّر] om. ELBOU || ٣ الثالثة عشر] الرابعة قال حبيش
U || ٦ وبخاصة] وبخاصّة EL || ٧ العطرة] العطرية ELBOU || ١٠ لثانية الأمراض
الحادة] في شرحه لتلك المقالة EL

(4) Fragrant seeds undo the harm of purgative[s] without hindering their action. Rather, they support their action, because they have the strength to cut and dilute the thick humors and to open the passages through which purgation takes place. *In Hippocratis De acutorum morborum [victu] et Galeni commentarius* 2.[5]

(5) Sometimes, when a purgative passes through the esophagus and cardia of the stomach, some of it sticks to these organs or settles in the stomach and causes great harm. Therefore, it is necessary to rinse these organs thereafter[6] by taking some barley gruel or barley groats. *In Hippocratis De acutorum morborum [victu] et Galeni commentarius* 2.[7]

(6) Says Moses: This rinsing should be done after the effect of the purgative has worn off but before the intake of soup of young chickens, so that the food does not mix with the residue of the purgative in the lining of the stomach. The rinsing should be done with a viscous substance that has a cleansing and moistening effect. For this reason, Hippocrates and Galen chose barley groats; and since they were used to this ingredient, it seemed fine to them to take a small amount of it, sufficient to rinse [the stomach] after the ingestion of the purgative. But if any of us would do so, he would quickly vomit the entire remedy. [Instead of that], it seems good to me to take a sip of hot julep. However, the consumption of barley groats, once the effect [of the purgative] has worn off, is something unusual in all the countries I have passed through. It causes nausea, because the stomach quickly needs to throw up [even] after the [effect of the] purgative [has worn off]. It seems to me that the best thing [to do] is to drink warm water in which marshmallow [*Althaea officinalis*] root or seed has been boiled together with fresh fennel [*Foeniculum vulgare*], or anise [*Pimpinella anisum*], or Chinese cinnamon [*Cinnamomum cassia* Nees], or the like in order to combine viscosity with that which has a cleansing effect and with fragrance and sweetness. This should be strained into sugar. If one adds myrtle [*Myrtus communis*][8] seed, it combines viscosity and fragrance. Moreover, it is a remedy which is good for the heart. Once this [compound medicine] leaves the stomach, eat the soup; and if the myrtle seed causes thirst, take fleawort [*Plantago psyllium* and var.] seed instead.

٤. البزور والعطرة تكسّر عادية الدواء المسهل ولا تمنعه من فعله بل تعينه على فعله لأنّ قوتها مقطعة ملطفة للأخلاط الغليظة مفتّحة للسبل الذي يكون بها الإسهال. في شرحه لثانية الأمراض الحادة.

٥. الدواء المسهل في ممرّه بالمرئ وفم المعدة قد يلصق بها منه شيء وربّما رسخ منه

٥ شيء في المعدة فيحدث ذلك ضررا عظيما. فلذلك ينبغي أن تغسل هذه الأعضاء بعده بتناول شيء من ماء الشعير أوكشكه. في شرحه لثانية الأمراض الحادة.

٦. قال موسى: ينبغي أن يكون هذا الغسل بعد انقضاء فعل الدواء قبل الاغتذاء بمرقة الفرّوج لئلا يخالط الغذاء تلك البقية التي بقيت من الدواء في خمل المعدة. وينبغي أن يكون الغسل بما فيه لزوجة وجلاء وترطيب. ولذلك اختار بقراط

١٠ وجالينوس كشك الشعير ولا اعتيادهما له حسن عندهما أن يتناول منه قدر يسير قدر ما يغسل بعقب الدواء. أمّا نحن فلو فعل أحدنا شيئا من ذلك لتقيّأ الدواء بجملته بسرعة. ويحسن عندي أن يتجرّع جرعة جلاب حارّ. وأمّا تناول كشك الشعير بعد انقضاء فعل الدواء فهو غير معتاد في عوائد جميع البلاد التي مرت بها ومغثّ لأنّ المعدة تسرع إلى تهوّع بعقب المسهل. وأجود ما يبدو لي أنه ينبغي أن يتناول ماء حارّ

١٥ قد أغلي فيه أصل خطمي أو بزره مع رازيانج أخضرا أو أنيسون أو دارصيني ونحوها ليجمع بين اللزوجة والجلاء والعطرية واللذاذة ويصفّى ذلك على سكّر. وإن ألقي عليه بزر ريحان فقد جمع بين اللزوجة والعطرية وهو دواء قلبي أيضا. فإذا خرج هذا عن المعدة يتناول المرق وإن وجد عطشا فيكون عوض بزر الريحان بزر قطونا.

---

١ العطرة] العطرية ELBOU | تكسّر] تفسد L | عادية] عادة B || ٤ يلصق] يلزق ELBOU | بها] بهما L || ٦ في شرحه لثانية الأمراض الحادة] في تلك المقالة EL || ٨ في خمل] فيدمل B || ٩ بقراط] ابقراط ELBOU || ١٠ ولا اعتيادهما] واعتيادهما G || ١١ بجملته] G¹ || ١٥ أغلي] غلي ELBOU

(7) In most cases, the evacuation by means of purgatives or emetics is not suitable. It is only necessary for someone with a drastic need for evacuation and should only be applied with long intervals [between uses]. *In Hippocratis Aphorismos commentarius* 3.[9]

(8) If you want to evacuate [the body] by means of a purgative or emetic, first dilute the thick humors, and cut the viscous ones, and widen the passages [using] a thinning regimen. If you want to purge [the body], first use a laxative for a number of times;[10] and if you want to apply emesis, first stimulate [the body] repeatedly.[11] *In Hippocratis Aphorismos Commentarius* 2.[12]

(9) Yellow bile can be evacuated with minimal effort. But phlegm— especially that which is very thick and viscous—and, equally, black bile can only be evacuated with difficulty. *De methodo [medendi]* 14.[13]

(10) All crude humors are slow to move because of their thickness and coldness. And once they move in order to be evacuated, they precede [the other superfluities] and close all the narrow passages. Therefore, do not use a purgative as long as there are crude, raw humors [in the body]. *De sanitate tuenda* 4.[14]

(11) Because of its thickness, one needs a stronger drug for the evacuation of black bile than for the evacuation of yellow bile. *In Hippocratis Aphorismos commentarius* 4.[15]

(12) For some people, it is sufficient to evacuate their body once a year at the beginning of spring. Others need a second evacuation in the fall. When bad humors have accumulated in the body, evacuate with drugs that cleanse the dominating [bad] humor. But when [large quantities of] superfluities have accumulated, evacuate them by venesection. *De sanitate tuenda* 6.[16]

(13) If you want to cleanse the body from the [bad] humors in it and, at the same time, want to cleanse the head so that no defluction descends from it, the remedy must be compounded from ingredients of varying

٧. الاستفراغ بالأدوية المسهلة أو المقيّئة ليس بموافقة في أكثر الأمر لأنّ هذا الاستفراغ إنّما يحتاج إليه من به حاجة شديدة إلى الاستفراغ وينبغي أن يكون فيما بين أوقات لها مدّة طويلة. في شرحه لثالثة الفصول.

٨. إذا أردت أن تستفرغ بدواء مسهل أو مقيّئ فتقدم ولطف الخلط الغليظ وقطع اللزج ووسع المجاري بالتدبير الملطف. فإن أردت الإسهال فلين البطن مرارا متوالية وإن كنت تريد أن تقيّئه فهيّج القيء مرارا كثيرة قبل ذلك. في شرحه لثانية الفصول.

٩. المرة الصفراء يسهل استفراغا بأهون سعي. وأمّا البلغم وخاصّة ما كان منه أغلظ وألزج وكذلك المرة السوداء فأنه عسر ما يستفرغ. آخر الحيلة.

١٠. الأخلاط النّيّة كلّها بطيئة الحركة لغلظها وبردها. فإذا حرّكت للاستفراغ سبقت فسدّت المجاري الضيّقة كلّها. وليس ينبغي أن يستعمل دواء مسهل ما دامت الأخلاط نيئة فجّة. رابعة تدبير الصحّة.

١١. يحتاج في استفراغ المرة السوداء إلى دواء أقوى ممّا يحتاج إليه في استفراغ الصفراء بسبب غلظها. في شرحه لرابعة الفصول.

١٢. بعض الناس يكتفي بأن يستفرغ بدنه مرة في السنة عند دخول الربيع وبعضهم يحتاج إلى استفراغ ثاني في الخريف. فإن كان المجتمع في البدن أخلاط رديئة فيستفرغ بالأدوية المنقية لذلك الخلط الغالب. فإن كان إنّما اجتمع فضل كثير فاستفرغه بالفصد. سادسة تدبير الصحّة.

١٣. إذا أردت أن تنقّي البدن ممّا فيه من الأخلاط وتنقّي الرأس معه حتّى لا تنزل منه نزلة فينبغي أن يكون الدواء مؤلّفا من أدوية مختلفة القوى بمنزلة الحبّ

٨ وأمّا] وبعدها L || ٩ فأنه] om. ELO || ١٧ فيستفرغ] فاستفرغ EL

strength—such as the pill I compounded from aloe [*Aloe vera*], scammony, pulp of the colocynth [*Citrullus colocynthis*], agaric [*Fomes officinalis*], blue bdellium [bdellium of *Balsamodendron africanum*] and gum [arabic]—because it expels many types of superfluities. If, at the end of
5   the treatment, one needs drugs to expel the black bile, use these.[17] *De methodo [medendi]* 5.[18]

(14) When one of the humors is completely evacuated from the body, it is necessarily affected by a bad temperament and a weakening of the vessels. The reason for such an evacuation cannot be attributed to a drug
10   alone but to an excessive purgation resulting from three things: one of these is the weakness of the vessels; the second, the wideness of the mouths of these vessels; and the third, the biting effect of the purgative. *De [simplicium] medicamentorum [temperamentis ac facultatibus]* 3.[19]

(15) If you administer a purgative, the first thing it expels is the
15   humor you intended to expel. If the purgation is excessive, the next thing to be expelled is the thinnest humor that remains, then the thickest, and then the blood. The thinnest humor is the yellow bile, followed by the phlegm, while the black bile is the thickest. However, blood comes last only once the drug overpowers nature and weakens its strength. *De*
20   *[simplicium] medicamentorum [temperamentis ac facultatibus]* 3.[20]

(16) Purgation becomes excessive if much of the strength of the [purgative] drug remains in the mouths of the vessels leading to the stomach. This then produces a biting in these vessels, and opens them, and constantly incites and stimulates them to expel their contents; it
25   also destroys the strength in the vessels. *De [simplicium] medicamentorum [temperamentis ac facultatibus]* 3.[21]

(17) If a person takes purgatives without any result, some of them have a bad effect, but others turn into food and do not harm his nature. These last-mentioned purgatives acquire strength from the body, through
30   which they attract and increase [so much] in purgative power that they turn into potential purgatives [again]. But if they do not realize that potential, they return to food. *De [simplicium] medicamentorum [temperamentis ac facultatibus]* 3.[22]

الذي ألّفناه نحن من صبر وسقمونيا وشثم حنظل وغاريقون ومقل أزرق وصمغ لأنه يخرج أنواعا كثيرة من أنواع الفضول. وإن احتجت في آخر الأمر إلى أدوية تخرج السوداء استعملها. خامسة الحيلة.

١٤. يجب ضرورة متى استفرغ من البدن واحد من الأخلاط كله جملة أن يعقب البدن منه سوء مزاج فتضعف العروق. والسبب في استفراغ ما ليس هو بخاصّي بالدواء بل لإفراط الإسهال بمحصوله في ثلاثة أشياء: أحدها ضعف العروق والثاني سعة أفواهها والثالث تلذيع الدواء المسهل. ثالثة الأدوية.

١٥. متى سقيت دواء مسهلا فأوّل ما يخرج ذلك الخلط الذي قصدت لإخراجه. فإن أفرط الإسهال خرج بعده أرقّ ما يبقى من الأخلاط ثم الأغلظ ثم الدم. وأرقّ الأخلاط الصفراء وبعدها البلغم والسوداء أغلظها. أما الدم فلا يأتي إلا أخيرا بعد أن يقهر الدواء الطبيعة ويوهن قواها. ثالثة الأدوية.

١٦. يفرط الإسهال عندما يبقى من الدواء قوة كثيرة في أفواه العروق التي تصير إلى المعدة فتحدث فيها لذعا وتفتحها وتحثها وتحرّكها إلى دفع ما فيها حثّا متصلا فتجحف بالقوة التي في العروق. ثالثة الأدوية.

١٧. إذا تناول الإنسان الأدوية المسهلة ولم تسهله فبعضها يؤثّر شرّا وبعضها يصير غذاء ليس على الطبيعة منه أذى وهي التي تكسب من البدن قوة تجذب بها وتزداد بتلك القوة إسهالا فكأنها مسهلة بالقوة. فإذا لم تخرج تلك القوة رجعت غذاء. ثالثة الأدوية.

١ وغاريقون] G¹ | وصمغ] om. G || ٦ بالدواء] G¹ || ٨ سقيت] أسقيت ELOU || ١٣ فتجحف] فتجحب EL || ١٥ يؤثّر] يورث EL: يؤثر شرّا وبعضها om. B || ١٧ إسهالا] إسهالها GU | فكأنها] فإنها ELO || ١٨ ثالثة الأدوية] في تلك المقالة EL

(18) I know famous physicians who are perplexed, not knowing what to do, when they administer purgatives that did not have any effect. When I am called in to such patients, I order some of them to bathe in the bathhouse, I prescribe venesection or emesis to others, and to [yet]

5   others [I apply] astringent remedies.[23] When I do this to them, their bowels become loose. *De [optimo] medico cognoscendo.*[24]

(19) It is necessary to bathe one, two, or three successive days before taking a cathartic remedy, because bathing melts the humors. When there is a site in the body that has become hard and tense, it becomes

10   softened and loose through the bathing, and the body becomes prepared so that [that] which streams through it does so in an easy way. *In Hippocratis Epidemiarum* 6.5.[25]

(20) Often, a single purgation is sufficient for curing those diseases that arise from yellow bile or phlegm. Those diseases which are more

15   related to black [bile], such as cancer and elephantiasis, cannot be cured by a single purgation, but need a second, third, fourth, or fifth [treatment]. *In Hippocratis De humoribus commentarius* 1.[26]

(21) The best therapy for someone in whom bile dominates is to evacuate him from below successively, on successive days. This should

20   be done both when he is healthy and when he is ill. *In Hippocratis Epidemiarum* 2.3.[27]

(22) When someone is disordered in his regimen[28] and addicted to drinking bad wines, you will not help him much by purging or phlebotomizing him, for crude humors quickly accumulate in his body in a

25   large amount because of his bad regimen. One should not undertake the treatment of such a patient at all. *De venae sectione.*[29]

١٨. وإني لأعلم قوما من مشهوري الأطباء يسقون دواء مسهلا فإذا لم يسهل بقوا حائرين لا يدرون ما يصنعون. وإذا دعينا لذلك أمرنا بعضهم بالاستحمام في الحمّام وفصدنا بعضهم وأمرنا بعضهم بالقيء وبعضهم بتناول شيء من الأدوية القابضة. فحين فعلنا ذلك بهم استطلقت بطونهم. في مقالته في محنة الطبيب.

٥

١٩. ينبغي الاستحمام قبل أخذ الدواء المنقّي بيوم ويومين وثلاثة متوالية لأنّ الاستحمام يذيب الأخلاط. وإن كان في البدن موضع قد صلب وتمدّد أرخاه وخلخله فيستعدّ البدن ليجري منه ما يجري بسهولة. في الخامسة من شرحه لسادسة أبيذيميا.

٢٠. ما كان من العلل من المرة الصفراء أو البلغم فكثيرا ما يجزّئ في برئها التنقية مرّة واحدة. وما كان أقرب إلى السوداء كالسرطان والجذام فليس يبرأ بالتنقية مرّة واحدة لكنّه ربّما احتاج إلى مرّة ثانية وثالثة ورابعة وخامسة. في شرحه للأولى من الأخلاط.

١٠

٢١. أجمل الأمور في من غلب عليه المرار أن يستفرغ منه مرارا متوالية في أيّام متوالية متّصلة من أسفل. ويفعل ذلك في حال الصحّة وفي حال المرض. في الثالثة من شرحه لثانية أبيذيميا.

١٥

٢٢. من كان مخلطا في تدبيره مغرى بشرب الشراب شربها ينتفع كثير منفعة إذا سقيته دواء مسهلا أو فصدته لأنّ الأخلاط النيئة تجتمع في بدنه كثيرا بسرعة لسوء تدبيره. ومن كان كذلك فلا ينبغي أصلا أن يقرب علاجه. في مقالته في الفصد.

Arabic translation, ed. Iskandar, الفاكهة [الأدوية ٣ || G¹ [بعضهم...بالاستحمام ٢

I.13 || أبيذيميا ELO [أبيديميا ٨ || التنقية B [السقية ٩ || بالتنقية B [السقية ١٠

om. G [مخلطا ١٦ || أبيذيميا ELOU [أبيديميا ١٥ || أجمع E [أجمل ١٣

(23) When you have a bowel movement, you should not interrupt it before the proper time, and when it stops by itself you should not leave it just like that.[30] Rather, examine and inspect the condition and quantity of the humors in the entire body. For when a small quantity remains, it causes a grave and dangerous illness. *In Hippocratis Epidemiarum* 2.1.[31]

(24) If you give a purgative to a patient, examine what is eliminated from him. If you observe that it has changed, know that his body is clean from the humor that you wanted to evacuate and he therefore benefits from this [treatment]. But this is not the case if the evacuated material consists of shreds,[32] or something bloodlike, or black bile, or something stinking, or a pure humor. For the excretion of humors in a pure state results from unnatural heat, and that of stinking material results from putrefaction, while that of black bile which is not quiescent[?][33] results from the prevailing burning.[34] *In Hippocratis Epidemiarum* 2.1.[35]

(25) Some people are hard to purge, while in others, a small quantity of a purgative effects a strong purgation. When the patient does not suffer from high fever and you know his nature, give him a purgative to drink. *De acutorum morborum [victu] et Galeni commentarius* 2.[36]

(26) The strength of a body that has been purged is weakened through the purgation. Therefore, it cannot tolerate much food nor digest it very well. Therefore, one should minimize a patient's food intake and increase it later on, slowly, and give him those foods which are quick to digest. *De acutorum morborum [victu] et Galeni commentarius* 2.[37]

٢٣. ليس ينبغي لك متى استطلق البطن أن تقطعه قبل الوقت الذي ينبغي ولا إن انقطع من تلقاء نفسه أن تدعه ينقطع. بل تتفقّد وتنظر كيف حال الأخلاط وما مقدارها في البدن كلّه فإنه إن بقي منها بقية ولّدت مرضا صعبا خطرا. في الأولى من شرحه لثانية أبيديميا.

٢٤. إذا سقيت دواء مسهلا فتأمّل ما يجيء صاحبه فإذا رأيت ما يجيء ه قد تغيّر فاعلم أنه قد نقي بدنه من الخلط الذي قصدت استفراغه ولذلك قد ينتفع به. إلا أن يكون الذي تغيّر إليه الاستفراغ خراطة أو شيء من جنس الدم أو سوداء أو شيء منتن أو خلط صرف لأن خروج الأخلاط صرفة من قبل حرارة خارجة عن الطبيعة والنتن من قبل العفونة وخروج السوداء التي لم تستودع لغلبة الاحتراق. في الأولى من شرحه لثانية أبيديميا.

٢٥. من الناس من يعسر إسهاله ومنهم من يسهله المقدار اليسير من الدواء إسهالا كثيرا. فمتى لم يكن بالمريض حتى قوية وكنت عارفا بطبيعته فاسقه دواء مسهلا. في شرحه لثانية الأمراض الحادة.

٢٦. قوة البدن الذي قد أسهل قد ضعفت بالإسهال ولذلك لا يمكنها احتمال الغذاء الكثير وتجويد هضمه. ولذلك ينبغي أن يقلّل من الغذاء ويزاد فيه في ما بعد على التدريج ويعطى من الأغذية ما كان سريع الانهضام. في شرحه لثانية الأمراض الحادة.

---

١ استطلق] استطلقت ELB || ٤ أبيديميا] أفيديميا ELOU || ٥ ما يجيء...طبيعته (٤٠) L om. || ٨ صرف] أصفر G || ٩ تستودع (= תמנה N) تستدع GU : تشرع O : (תמהר Z=) تستعر G || que non greditur Bo E(?) || ١٥ ويزاد...سريع] G¹

(27) If a very high fever develops, be extremely careful not to administer a purgative. Evacuate especially through bloodletting, because evacuation by means of bloodletting does not involve any danger. *De acutorum morborum [victu] et Galeni commentarius* 2.[38]

(28) When diarrhea is beneficial, one should not interrupt it—not even with food that only has little binding force, and certainly not with binding drugs. For if it is interrupted, the bad humor reascends, and a fever or tumor develops in the liver,[39] usually, or in another organ. *In Hippocratis Epidemiarum* 2.2.[40]

(29) When you intend to administer a purgative, be especially[41] careful during [fever] attacks or critical days. The strength of the purgative is corrupted if the humors tend toward the upper parts of the body or to the side opposite from where the drug evacuates them. *In Hippocratis De humoribus commentarius* 2.[42]

(30) I have cured countless patients who suffered from jaundice by [using] purgation only. Similarly, I have cured those who suffered from elephantiasis or from a chronic and long-standing pain and from other chronic illnesses by purgation alone. *De [optimo] medico cognoscendo.*[43]

(31) Many people are quick to find relief and to rejoice at a strong evacuation. But the more they are evacuated on the first day, the more constipated they are on the following days. *De sanitate tuenda* 5.[44]

(32) When we want to purge infants, we give their wetnurses something from a purgative to drink, for the strength of that [purgative] stays in the milk. That this is so is evident from other living creatures, for the bowels of some people were relieved from drinking the milk of goats that had fed on the branches of scammony or latex plants. Others ate a lot of

٢٧. متى حدثت حمّى قوية جدًّا فاحذر حذرا شديدا من إسقاء دواء مسهل واستفرغ بالفصد خاصّة لأنّ الاستفراغ بالفصد ليس يقع فيه شيء من الخطر. في شرحه لثانية الأمراض الحادّة.

٢٨. الاختلاف إذا كان ينتفع به فلا ينبغي أن يقطع ولو بالطعام الذي معه قوة يسيرة من الحبس فضلا عن الأدوية الحابسة، فإنّه إن قطع عاد الخلط الرديء إلى فوق وولد حمّى أو ورم في الكبد على الأكثر أو في سائر الأعضاء. في ثانية من شرحه لثانية أبيديميا.

٢٩. ينبغي لك أن تحذر متى هممت بإعطاء دواء مسهل بكثرة أوقات النوائب أو أيّام البحارين. وذلك أنّ قوة الدواء تفسد إذا كان ميل الأخلاط إلى أعالي البدن أو إلى ضدّ الجهة التي يستفرغ بها الدواء. في ثانية من شرح الأخلاط.

٣٠. لا أحصي كم من عليل كان به يرقان أبرأته بالإسهال فقط. وكذلك من كان به جذام أو ألم مزمن متقادم وغير ذلك من الأمراض المزمنة أبرأته بالإسهال فقط. في مقالته في محنة الطبيب.

٣١. كثير من الناس يستريحون في عاجل الأمر إلى الاستفراغ القوي ويسرّون به. وبحسب كثرة ما يستفرغ منه في أول يوم يكون احتباس الطبيعة فيما بعد من الأيّام. خامسة تدبير الصحّة.

٣٢. إذا أردنا أن نسهل الأطفال سقينا مرضعاتهم شيئا من الأدوية المسهلة فقوة ذلك باقية في لبنها. وذلك بيّن في سائر الحيوان فإنّ قوما انسهلت بطونهم من شرب لبن ماعز ارتعت أغصان سقمونيا أو يتوع. وقوم أكثروا من أكل السمّان

---

quails and were affected by tension in the muscles because of the hellebore [*Helleborus albus* var. *niger*] on which the quails fed. *In Hippocratis
Epidemiarum librum* 6.5.[45]

(33) One should apply an enema only to someone whose strength is
great. But in the case of someone whose strength is weak, one should use
a suppository. *De acutorum morborum [victu] et Galeni commentarius* 3.[46]

(34) Some ancient physicians recommend that someone suffering
from a colic take a small stone of salt and use it as a suppository, because
it expels the excrements in a light and easy way. Natron may have the
same effect if used as a suppository. *De colica.*[47]

(35) If one takes two parts of tar and one part of olive oil and applies
it as an enema, it is very beneficial for a colic, when the stomach is
strong. But when the stomach of the patient is weak, avoid it. Similarly,
other strong medications should be applied as enemas only when the
stomach is strong. When the patient has a weak stomach, he should be
given only enemas with mild medications, so that the stomach does not
weaken even more and the patient does not get one disease after the
other. For when strong medications are applied as an enema, the strength
of the enema sometimes reaches the stomach and may, [from there],
even reach up to the tongue. *De colica.*

(36) If there are biting moistures in the intestines, one should, first
of all, apply an enema with something that washes them, such as
hydromel or barley gruel. And once they have been expelled from the
intestines, [one should apply an enema] with that whose property it is
to alleviate the biting [pain] and to have an agglutinant and cohesive
effect. *In Hippocratis Epidemiarum* 6.6.[48]

(37) We use an enema with salt water in the case of someone who
suffers from putrid ulcers in his intestines, so that it washes all that had
putrefied and expels a substantial amount of scales.[49] Once the site is
clean, we apply an enema with drugs that are good for the putrefaction.[50]
In Hippocratis De humoribus commentarius 1.[51]

واعتراهم تمدد في العضل من قبل الحريق الذي رعته السمّان. في خامسة من شرحه لسادسة أبيديميا.

٣٣. إنّما ينبغي أن تحقن من قوته قوية وأمّا من قوته ضعيفة فاستعمل فيه الفتيلة. من شرحه لثالثة الأمراض الحادّة.

٣٤. وقد كان بعض القدماء يأمر من أصابه القولنج أن يأخذ حجرا صغيرا من ملح فيحتمله فإنه يخرج النجو خروجا سهلا سريعا. وقد يفعل ذلك النطرون إذا احتمل. في مقالته في القولنج.

٣٥. إذا أخذ من القطران جزءان ومن الزيت جزء واحتقن به نفع من القولنج منفعة عظيمة إن كانت المعدة قوية. أمّا إن كانت معدة العليل ضعيفة فاجتنبه. وكذلك استعمال سائر الأدوية القوية في الحقن لا يفعل إلا إن كانت المعدة قوية. أمّا المعدة الضعيفة فلا يحقن صاحبها إلا بالأدوية اللينة لئلا تزيد المعدة ضعفا وينتقل العليل من مرض إلى مرض لأن الأدوية القوية إذا احتقن بها ربّما بلغ عظم الحقنة إلى المعدة ويرقى إلى اللسان. في مقالته في القولنج.

٣٦. إذا كانت رطوبات لذّاعة في المعاء فينبغي أن يحقن أوّلا بما يغسله مثل ماء العسل وماء الشعير فإذا خرجت فاحقن بما شأنه أن يسكّن اللذع وبما من شأنه أن يغري ويلصق. في السادسة من شرحه لسادسة أبيديميا.

٣٧. الحقنة بماء الملح قد نستعملها من كان في أمعائه قروح عفنة فتغسل كلّ ما كان قد عفن وتخرج قشورا ليست بالصغار. وإذا نقي الموضع حقنا بالأدوية التي تصلح العفونة. في شرحه لأولى من الأخلاط.

---

٨ به] بذلك EBOU || ١١ الضعيفة] G[1] || ١٦ ويلصق] ويلزق EBOU | أبيديميا] أبيفيميا OU

(38) As much as possible, one should be careful and considerate concerning the other types of evacuation[52] in the case of someone whose bodily condition is such that his flesh is soft and slack, lean, and quick to dissolve. Similarly, [one should take care] in the case of someone who is extremely fat or lean. Such a person should be, first of all, evacuated by means of a moderate diet, massage, mild enemas, the application of fomentations and poultices and softening suppositories, and bathing. Be careful to apply these [means] according to the indications provided by the conditions of the patient. *Ad Glauconem [de methodo medendi]* 1.[53]

(39) For ulcerous wombs, we often apply enemas with milk boiled with stones or iron. We also provide benefit [with this remedy] in the case of hemorrhoids and ulcers in the anus. *De [simplicium] medicamentorum [temperamentis ac facultatibus]* 10.[54]

(40) If you need to apply an enema for someone with constipation, be it someone who has a chronic disease or someone on a diet of a convalescent after a lengthy disease, do not use a sharp enema, but one containing olive oil only. *De sanitate tuenda* 5.[55]

(41) One should attempt to relieve the bowels of someone suffering from a continuous putrid fever; and if his bowels cannot be relieved, one should give the patient an enema with hydromel and olive oil. *De methodo [medendi]* 11.[56]

(42) When biting humors incline toward the intestines, evacuate them by administering the patient an enema from below with an appropriate ingredient. The best and most appropriate ingredient is barley gruel. *De methodo [medendi]* 12.[57]

(43) The enemas to be used for intestinous ulcers should be composed from astringent, cleansing, ripening, stupefying, agglutinant, and alleviating ingredients. If you intend [to use an enema with] one of these effects, or all of them, or whichever is needed, then the base for these medications should be barley gruel and some astringent wine. Use this for an enema. *Mayāmir* 9.[58]

٣٨. ينبغي أن يستعمل القصد والتوقّي ما أمكن في سائر أنواع الاستفراغ ممّن كانت حالة بدنه أن يكون له لينا رخوا سخيفا سريع التحلّل. وكذلك من أفرط عليه السمن أو الهزال. ويكون استفراغه أوّلا بالحمية المعتدلة والدلك والحقن اللينة والتنطيل والتضميد وباحتمال الأشياف المليّنة وبالحمّام. تقصد من هذه بحسب ما

٥ تدلّك عليه أحوال المريض. في أولى أغلوقن.

٣٩. كثيرا ما نحقن الأرحام ذوات القروح بهذا اللبن المطبوخ بالحجارة والحديد وننفع به البواسير والقروح الحادثة في المقعدة. عاشرة الأدوية.

٤٠. إذا احتجت في من احتبست طبيعته ممّن به مرض مزمن أو ممن يدبّر تدبير الناقه بعد طول من المرض إلى استعمال حقنة لم تستعمل منها ما هو حادّ، بل احقن

١٠ بالزيت وحده. خامسة تدبير الصحّة.

٤١. يقصد إطلاق بطن المحمومين حتّى مطبقة عفنية وإن لم ينطلق البطن فيحقن العليل بماء عسل وزيت. حادية عشر الحيلة.

٤٢. إذا مالت أخلاط لذاعة إلى الأمعاء فاستفرغها بأن تحقن المريض من أسفل بشيء موافق. وأفضل هذه الأشياء وأولاها ماء كشك الشعير. ثانية عشر الحيلة.

٤٣. الحقن التي تحقن بها لقرحة الأمعاء تؤلّف من أمور قابضة ومنقّية ومنضجة

١٥ ومخدّرة ومغرية ومسكّنة. أمّا إن تقصد أحد هذه الأغراض أو كلّها أو ما دعت الحاجة إليه وتجعل مادّة تلك الأدوية ماء كشك الشعير ويسير شراب قابض ويحقن بها. تاسعة الميامر.

---

٩ إلى] على EBOU | بل] لكن EBOU || ١١ يقصد...حادية عشر الحيلة] om. B

(44) Rules in hortatory form[59] composed by Abū al-ʿAlāʾ ibn Zuhr[60]
for his son Abū Marwān[61] concerning the treatment [by means of] purgatives which every physician should observe—all of them. He said: "Be
most careful not to administer strong purgatives [initially], but begin
5   with cocting [the humors], opening the obstructions, washing the passages, and softening the stool. Then you can purge. When it is necessary
to purge the bowels during the cold season, one should mix with the purgatives [substances] that dissolve the humors, such as the [different] kinds
of salt and long pepper [*Piper longum*]. If you are forced to purge during
10   the hot season, you do not need a dissolving [substance]. In any case, it is
necessary to use, in combination with the purgative, a [substance] that
strengthens the stomach, such as mastic [resin of *Pistacia lentiscus*], anisc,
[or] absinthe [*Artemisia absinthium* and var.]; and [a substance] that hinders
[the purgative] from passing from the intestines into the liver and that
15   protects against its harmful effects, such as almonds [*Prunus amygdalis*
var. *amara* var. *dulcis*] and pistachios [*Pistacia vera* and var.] and their oils,
or a rob[62] of licorice [*Glycyrrhiza glabra*], or gum tragacanth [resin of several species of *Astragalus*], and or the like."

(45) He further said: "The more one washes purgatives, the more
20   one diminishes their purgative effect. The same applies if one boils them.
The more one pulverizes them, the more likely they are to be lethal
rather than purgative. When they are safe, they induce micturition. But
all astringent things act conversely. The more one washes or boils them,
the more astringent they become. Similarly, the more one pulverizes
25   them, the more astringent they become, and they also hold back the urine."

(46) He further said: "Any purgative with which you want to purify
the head should be administered in the form of large pills and should
have a strong effect. When he goes to bed, the patient should take such
a purgative with hot water in which raisins have been cooked until they
30   rise. Always add a little garlic [*Allium sativum*] to any medication [used]
for purifying the head."

٤٤. لأبي العلاء بن زهر وصايا لابنه أبي مروان في تدبير الأدوية المسهلة ينبغي أن يتدبّرها الطبيب كلّها وهي هذه قال: يتحفّظ جدّا من إعطاء الأدوية القوية الإسهال ويتقدّم أيضا بالإنضاج وتفتيح السدد وغسل المجاري وتليين الطبع وحينئذ يسهل. وإن دعت الضرورة لإسهال البطن في زمان البرد فيخلط في

٥ المسهلات ما يذيب الأخلاط كأنواع الملح والدارفلفل. فإن اضطررت للإسهال في زمان حرّ فلا حاجة إلى ما يذيب. وفي كلّ حال لا بدّ مع الدواء المسهل ممّا يقوّي المعدة كالمصطكى وأنيسون وأفسنتين وما يحجب بين الأمعاء والكبد وبين نكاية المسهلات كاللوز والفستق ودهنهما وربّ السوس وكثيراء ونحوها.

٤٥. من كلامه: كلّ المسهلات كلّما نقص إسهالها وكذلك إن أغليتها.

١٠ وكلّما بالغت في سحقها كانت أولى بأن تقتل منها بأن تسهل منها. وإن كانت مأمونة أدرّت البول. وكلّ المقبّضات بالضدّ، كلّما غسلتها أو أطلت طبخها ازدادت قبضا. وكذلك كلّما سحقتها زادت قبضا وإمساك للبول أيضا.

٤٦. من كلامه: كلّ مسهل تريد به تنقية الرأس تحبّه كبارا ويكون في الحبوب شدّة. وناوله عند النوم بماء حارّ قد أغلي فيه زبيب حتّى يرقى إلى فوق. واخلط

١٥ أبدا يسيرمن الثوم في الدواء المنقّي للرأس.

---

٩ أغليتها] غليتها ELBU || ١٤ أغلي] غلي ELBOU

(47) He further said: "Imagine a boy who is stricken by a fever that dissolves his flesh to the degree that it comes out in the diarrhea. The most effective way to stop the diarrhea is to immerse the patient in cold water. Imagine someone with coarse humors who is given a purgative

5   while the weather is cold, for he suffers from distress and disturbance and pains in the stomach and intestines, but does not respond to the medicine. If you let him go to the bathhouse and he goes into a hot bathing basin, in due time his bowels will be relieved and his humors will respond and leave [his body], and his pains and distress will be

10   alleviated. And if someone with thin humors who is given a [purgative] drug while the weather is cold and who, consequently, suffers from severe diarrhea goes into a hot bathing basin in the bathhouse, his diarrhea will stop. In the first [case], the [heat of the] bath dissolves and expels his [coarse] humors; while in the second [case], the heat of the

15   bath attracts the humors to the outside."[63]

(48) He further said: "There are [certain] purgatives that have no effect on [certain] individuals, while a medication that is weaker does have a [certain therapeutic] effect on them. If you give a medication and it does not have any effect, do not give more [of the same], but give

20   a different one, even if it is less potent, be it [some] days after the initial medication or shortly thereafter. Never allow a patient to eat immediately after taking a purgative. Let him take light food before [the ingestion] of the purgative and afterwards for [some] days, according to the strength of the drug."

25   (49) He further said: "It is a mistake to use musk as a part of purgatives, and, similarly, to drink it with wine. Those who compound this remedy [and administer it] are mistaken, because they want to strengthen the organs and let the medicine rise to the head; but [they] forget that the effect of these purgatives is carried to the major organs, and sometimes

30   such an organ cannot tolerate this, and [the patient] is killed."

(50) Says Moses: This is correct if the purgation is done by poisonous drugs, such as pulp of colocynth or turbith [*Ipomoea turpethum*], because of their poisonous effect; or [by strong drugs, such as] laurel [*Laurus nobilis*], because of its strength. But safe drugs—and especially agaric,

35   which is good for poisons—are very beneficial if imbibed in wine. I have done so several times [and used such a drug] in order to cleanse the head, and [I] saw that it is very effective and that it cleanses the brain to a degree any [other] drug is incapable of. Moreover, the patient taking this drug found [new] energy and dilation of the soul. Therefore, con-

40   sider the specific properties of the drugs that you administer.

٤٧. من كلامه: تخيّل شابّاً أصابته حتى تذيب له فيخرج بالإسهال. فأبلغ شيئاً في قطع هذا الإسهال أن يغمس العليل في الماء البارد. وتخيّل من سقي دواء مسهلاً وأخلاطه غليظة والهواء بارد فإنّه يحدث له كرب واضطراب وأوجاع في المعدة والأمعاء ولا يجيب الدواء. فإذا أدخلته الحمّام ونزل في الأبزن الحارّ فلحينه ينطلق بطنه وتجيب أخلاطه للخروج وتسكن أوجاعه وكربه. أمّا من كانت أخلاطه رقيقة وسقي الدواء والهواء بارد فأفرط إسهاله فإنّه عند نزوله في الأبزن الحارّ في الحمّام يرتفع إسهاله. أمّا الأوّل فإنّ الحمّام أذاب أخلاطه فأطلقها والثاني جذبها حرّ الحمّام إلى خارج.

٤٨. من كلامه: في الأدوية المسهلة ما لا يؤثّر في أفراد من الناس ويؤثّر فيهم دواء دون تلك الأدوية في القوة. فإن سقيت دواء ولم يؤثّر فلا تزيد منه بل اسق غيره وإذا ضعف من قوته إمّا بعد أيّام من الدواء الأوّل أو بالقرب منه. ولا تجمع أبداً بين المسهل والغذاء ولطف الغذاء قبل المسهل وبعده بأيّام بحسب قوة الدواء.

٤٩. من كلامه: استعمال المسك في الأدوية المسهلة وكذلك شربها بالخمر خطأ. ووهم وقع لمن ركّب ذلك لأنّهم قصدوا تقوية الأعضاء وسمو الدواء إلى الرأس ونسوا ما يحتمله من قوة الأدوية المسهلة إلى الأعضاء الرئيسة فيّما لم يحتمله ذلك العضو فقتل.

٥٠. قال موسى: هذا صحيح إذا كان الإسهال بأدوية سميّة أو قوية كسمّ الحنظل والتربد لسميّتها أو الرند لقوته. وأمّا الأدوية المأمونة وبخاصّة الغاريقون الذي هو دواء ينفع من السموم فما أنفع سقيه بالخمر. فقد فعلت ذلك مرّات لتنقية الرأس فرأيت له فعلاً عظيماً ونقّى الدماغ تنقية عجز عنها كلّ دواء. ووجد شاربه نشاطاً وبسط نفس. فاعتبر خواصّ الأدوية التي تسقيها.

١٣ الأعضاء] G¹ || ١٦ كان] G¹ | الإسهال] U¹ : ELO om. || ١٨ من] G¹ || ١٩ فعلاً] أثراً ELBOU | ووجد] ويجد L

(51) He further said: [In the case of] the rind [enclosing] the pulp of colocynth and kernels of pistachio, followed by almond kernels, this[64] has been confirmed by long experience. [The same applies to] husks of hellebore [*Helleborus*] [and] nenuphar [*Nymphae*] blossoms. And if one adds almond oil thereto, it is a good decision.

(52) In his [book entitled] *Al-murshid*, al-Tamīmī[65] states: "If one boils milk and adds thereto—when it boils—seeds of garden cress [*Lepidium sativum*], without pulverizing them, and lets this boil until the mucilage emerges, and then one drinks this milk, it cures the colics resulting from taking purgatives, whether pills or decoctions. One should drink [the milk] while it is lukewarm, because it has a glutinous effect on the [contents of] the intestines and [at the same time] washes the remainder of the purgative from the stomach and the intestines."

(53) Says Moses: This is correct on the condition that one uses goat's milk. And if the patient who takes the medicine becomes very thirsty and feels burning in the stomach and intestines, [the ingestion of] fleawort seed with cold water and rose syrup is most appropriate.

(54) In his [book entitled] *Al-murshid*, al-Tamīmī further states that, because of its specific properties, an onion [*Allium cepa*], when one crushes it and smells it during the ingestion of a purgative, stops the nausea and prevents the purgative from being vomited.

This is the end of the thirteenth treatise,
by the grace of God, praise be to Him.

◆

٥١. من كلامه: حجاب شم الحنظل لب الفستق وبعده لب اللوز صح ذلك بتجربة طويلة .
وحجاب الحريق زهر النيلوفر وإن انضاف إلى ذلك دهن اللوز كان ذلك من الحزم .

٥٢. ذكر التيمي في المرشد إذا أغلي اللبن وألقي فيه في حال غليانه حب رشاد غير
مسحوق وأغلي حتى يخرج لعابه فيه فإن شرب ذلك اللبن يشفي من الأمغاص الكائنة
بعقب شرب الأدوية المسهلة حبوبا كانت أو مطبوخات . ويشرب وهو فاتر ويغري
الأمعاء ويغسل بقايا الدواء من المعدة والأمعاء .

٥٣. قال موسى: هذا صحيح ويشترط أن يكون لبن ماعز . وإن وجد شارب
الدواء عطشا شديدا وتلهبا في المعدة والأمعاء فإن بزر قطونا بماء بارد وشراب
ورد أوفق في هذه الحال .

٥٤. وذكر التيمي في المرشد أن البصل إذا شدخ وشم عند شرب الدواء المسهل
قطع الغثيان ومنع قذفه بخاصية فيه .

تمت المقالة الثالث عشر ولله الحمد والمنة .

---

٣ المرشد] أنّه .add EL : أنّ OU || أغلي] غلي EBOU || ٤ أغلي] غلي ELBOU ||
٥ حبوبا كانت أو مطبوخات] G¹ || ٦ الأمعاء] المعاء G || ٧ ويشترط] في اللبن .add
ELBOU || ٨ بارد] om. ELBOU | وشراب] وبشراب U : وبشراب أو بشراب O ||
١٢ تمت المقالة الثالثة عشر ولله الحمد والمنة] تمت المقالة الثالثة عشر والحمد لله كثيرا E : تمت
المقالة وعدد فصولها أربعة وخمسين فصلا L : تمت المقالة B : كملت المقالة وعدد فصولها أربعة
وخمسين فصلا والحمد لواهب العقل O : تمت المقالة الثامنة لحبيش والحمد لله عدد فصولها خمسين U

In the name of God,
the Merciful, the Compassionate.
O Lord, make [our task] easy

The Fourteenth Treatise

Containing aphorisms concerning vomiting

(1) All the phlegm that streams into the intestines or that originates in it is washed by the yellow bile superfluity and excreted in the stool. Sometimes much phlegm also originates in the stomach, and therefore the ancient physicians advised [that] once every month, [one should] induce vomiting after [taking] food. Some of them thought that one should vomit twice [a month]. All of them advised that the food taken prior to vomiting should have a sharp taste and a cleansing and detergent strength, in order to clean all the phlegm out of the stomach without the body being harmed by a bad [condition of the humors] originating from [such food]; because all detergent, biting foods produce yellow bile, and all of them are unwholesome. *De usu partium* 5.[1]

بسم الله الرحمن الرحيم

ربّ يسّر

المقالة الرابعة عشر

تشتمل على فصول تتعلّق بالقيء

١. كلّ ما ينصبّ من البلغم إلى الأمعاء أو يتولّد فيها فإنّ فضلة المرّة الصفراء ٥
تغسله وتخرجه مع الغائط. والمعدة أيضًا قديمًا تولّد فيها بلغم كثير ولذلك أشار القدماء
من الأطبّاء باستعمال القيء بعد الطعام في كلّ شهر مرّة واحدة. وبعضهم رأى أنّه
ينبغي أن يتقيّأ مرّتين. وجميعهم يشير بأن يكون ما يتناول من الأغذية قبل القيء ما كان
حرّيف الطعم ذا قوّة تجلو وتغسل لكيما ينقّي جميع ما في المعدة من البلغم من غير أن تضرّ
بالبدن رداءة ما يتولّد عنها لأنّ الأغذية الغسّالة اللذّاعة تولّد جميعها مرّة صفراء ١٠
وكلّها رديئة الغذاء. خامسة المنافع.

---

١ بسم الله الرحمن الرحيم ربّ يسّر [om. ELBOU || ٣ المقالة الرابعة عشر] المقالة الخامسة
قال حبيش U || ٥ إلى الأمعاء] للأمعاء ELBOU || ١١ خامسة] خامسة عشر B

(2) If someone's body contains sharp, biting humors,[2] one should not induce vomiting for fear that some of the external superfluities retreat inward; for one should be cautious not to attract the biting humors to the inside, just as one should be cautious not to drive the raw humors which surround the liver to the outside. *De sanitate tuenda* 4.[3]

(3) Melancholic humors should always be evacuated from below and not through vomiting at all. [Thus he said] in his commentary to *De humoribus* 1.[4] And in his *Commentary on Aphorisms* 4,[5] he said that if a sharp, thin humor floats upward, there is no way to evacuate it through vomiting in wintertime.

(4) If someone is stricken by syncope because of bad humors that irritate the cardia of his stomach, give him hot, pure water to drink, [either alone] or mixed with some oil. Then tell him to vomit; but if vomiting is too difficult for him, warm his stomach and its adjacent parts and his feet and hands. But if, even in this way, vomiting does not come to him, induce it by entering your finger or a feather [into his throat]. But if, even then, vomiting does not come to him, give him the best oil that you can dispose of to drink, heated. But in many cases, this oil has the property not to induce vomiting, but to soften the stool.[6] And this is also beneficial for someone suffering from this condition. *Ad Glauconem [De methodo medendi]* 1.[7]

(5) When bilious humor tends upward to the stomach, evacuate it through vomiting after exercise but prior to [taking] food. To apply vomiting is most appropriate in the case of someone whose temperament tends more toward heat and dryness since the beginning of the [illness]. *De sanitate tuenda* 6.[8]

(6) If someone's stomach contains viscous phlegm that fills it completely, and [if] he is one of those who vomit easily, he will come to no harm if he vomits by means of radish [*Raphanus sativus* and var.] with oxymel. If the phlegm is thin and not viscous, barley gruel alone or

٢. من كان في بدنه أخلاط حادّة لذّاعة فلا ينبغي أن يستعمل القيء خوفا من أن يتراجع شيء من الفضول التي خارج إلى داخل لأنه ينبغي أن يحذر جذب الأخلاط اللذّاعة إلى داخل كما يتّقى جذب الأخلاط النيئة التي حول الكبد إلى خارج. رابعة تدبير الصحّة.

٣. الخلط السوداوي ينبغي أن تستفرغه دائما من أسفل ولا تستفرغه بالقيء بتّة. في شرحه للأولى من الأخلاط. وقال في شرحه لرابعة الفصول إنه لو كان الخلط حادّا لطيفا يطفو إلى فوق فلا سبيل إلى استفراغه بالقيء إذا كان الوقت شتاء.

٤. من يصيبه الغشي بسبب أخلاط رديئة تلذع فم معدته فاسقه ماء حارّا قراحا أو مخلوطا بشيء من الأدهان، ثمّ مره بالقيء فإن كان القيء يعسر عليه فسخّن معدته ونواحيها وقدميه وكفّيه. فإن لم يطاوعه القيء ولا بهذا فهيّج القيء بإدخال الإصبع أو الريشة. فإن لم يطاوعه القيء ولا بهذا فاسقه دهنا أجود ما تقدر عليه مسخنا. ومن شأن هذا الدهن في كثير من الحالات أن لا يهيّج القيء بل يليّن الطبيعة ولذلك أيضا لصاحب هذه الحال صلاح. أولى أغلوقن.

٥. متى كان ميل الخلط الصفراوي إلى فوق نحو المعدة فاجعل استفراغه بالقيء بعد الرياضة قبل الطعام. وأحرى باستعمال القيء من كان مزاجه منذ أول الأمر أميل ألى الحرارة واليبس. سادسة تدبير الصحّة.

٦. من كان في معدته بلغم لزج يستغرقها وكان ممن يسهل عليه القيء فلا بأس بأن يتقيّأ بفجل مع سكنجبين. وإن كان بلغما رقيقا غير لزج فماء كشك الشعير وحده أو

٣ يتّقى] توق EOU || ٥ بتّة] البتّة EOU || ٨ فاسقه] فاسقيه G || ١٠ فهيّج... ولا بهذا] om. ELBO || ١٢ ولذلك] وفي ذلك ELBOU || ١٤ الخلط الصفراوي] الأخلاط الصفراوية ELB || ١٧ بأس بأن] G¹

hydromel alone is sufficient to induce vomiting, when one takes, of either one of these, a dose larger than that which one would take in order to feed oneself with it. *De methodo [medendi]* 6.[9]

(7) If you want to let someone vomit after a meal, feed him brains seasoned with much olive oil after his meal, because this induces vomiting. *De alimentorum [facultatibus]* 3.[10]

(8) The bulb of the narcissus [*Narcissus*] is one of the drugs that induces vomiting. Therefore, we add two or three bulbs to the food of someone in whom we want to induce vomiting, for then he will vomit easily, without any harm. *In Hippocratis Epidemiarum* 2.6.[11]

(9) If it is easy for someone to vomit, he should do so before [taking] food, in order to cleanse his body from the superfluities of the [previous] food [he took]. If it is difficult for someone to vomit, he should vomit after [taking] food, in order to cleanse his body from the phlegm as well. *In Hippocratis De mulierum affectibus commentarius.*[12]

(10) He [Galen] said: "Vomiting can often be applied for cleansing a thick, viscous humor which has settled in the stomach. And there is no hindrance in either one of these cases from vomiting on all days, but they should not apply it on two successive days only." *In Hippocratis De natura hominis commentarius.*[13]

(11) If someone's stomach contains biting humors that either originate there or pour [into it] and [if] he is nearly fainting, let him vomit by giving him lukewarm water to drink. *De methodo [medendi]* 12.[14]

(12) Heavy movement of the body after the imbibition of an emetic helps vomiting, because the movement stimulates the humors upwards, as happens to sailors. *In Hippocratis Aphorismos commentarius* 4.[15]

ماء العسل وحده يكفيه القيء به إذا تناول من أحدهما قدراً أكثر مما يتناول ليغتذي به. سابعة الحيلة.

٧. متى أردت أن تستدعي من إنسان القيء بعد الطعام فاطعمه بعد طعامه دماغاً قد طيّب بزيت كثير فإنه يهيّج بالقيء. ثالثة الأغذية.

٨. بصل النرجس من الأدوية المهيّجة للقيء ولذلك نطعم من أردنا أن نقيّئه منها بصلتين أو ثلاثة مع طعامه فإنه يتقيأ بسهولة من غير أذى. سادسة شرحه لثانية أبيديميا.

٩. من كان القيء يسهل عليه فيستعمل القيء قبل الطعام لينقّي بدنه من فضول الطعام. ومن كان القيء يعسر عليه فينبغي أن يتقيأ بعد الطعام لينقّي أيضاً بدنه من البلغم. في شرحه لأوجاع النساء.

١٠. قال: كثيراً ما يستعمل القيء لتنقية خلط غليظ لزج قد رسخ في المعدة وليس يمنع مانع لأحد من هؤلاء أن يستعمل القيء في الأيام كلّها ولا يستعملون يومين متوالين فقط. في شرحه لطبيعة الإنسان.

١١. متى كان في المعدة أخلاط لذّاعة تتولّد هناك أو تنصبّ ويقارب صاحبها الغشي فاستعمل القيء بأن تجرعه ماء فاتراً. ثانية عشر الحيلة.

١٢. تحريك البدن حركة ثقيلة بعد شرب المقيئ مما يعين على القيء لأن الحركة تثير الأخلاط إلى فوق كما يعتري ركّاب السفن. في شرحه لرابعة الفصول.

---

١ وحده] وهذا L ‖ ٢ سابعة] في الأول L ‖ ٧ أبيديميا] أفيديميا ELOU ‖ ٨ فيستعمل...عليه] G¹: فيستعمل] ليستعمل EL | فضول] فضل G ‖ ١١ قال] G¹ ‖ ١٦ ثقيلة] نقلة EGLOU

(13) Drugs that induce vomiting should not be taken all at once but little by little, so that they stay in the stomach and dissolve and attenuate. Then one should take a larger dose until the moment that all that is in the stomach and in the main adjacent vessels is evacuated. *In Hippocratis De natura hominis commentarius.*[16]

5

This is the end of the fourteenth treatise,
by the grace of God, praise be to Him.

◆

١٣. الأشياء التي يتقيأ بها ينبغي أن لا تؤخذ دفعة إلا شيء بعد شيء ورفق حتى تلبث في المعدة وتقطع وتلطف. وبعد ذلك يزاد في الشرب حتى يستفرغ ما في المعدة وما في العروق الأول التي تليها. في شرحه لطبيعة الإنسان.

تمّت المقالة الرابعة عشر ولله الحمد والمنة.

---

١ تؤخذ] G¹ ‖ ٤ تمّت المقالة الرابعة عشر ولله الحمد والمنة] تمّت المقالة الرابعة عشر والحمد لله كثيرا E : تمّت المقالة وعدد فصولها ثلاثة عشر فصلا L تمّت المقالة B : كلّت المقالة الرابعة عشر وعدد فصولها ثلاثة عشر والحمد لله O : تمّت المقالة السادسة عدد فصولها ثلاث عشر U

In the name of God,
the Merciful, the Compassionate.
O Lord, make [our task] easy

The Fifteenth Treatise

Containing aphorisms concerning surgery

(1) Putrid ulcers that spread and expand to the surrounding area require very strong remedies. From time to time, cauterization is needed as part of their treatment. *Qāṭājānas* 5.[1]

(2) Some ulcers are called carbuncles. The site where they occur looks as if [it has been] burned by fire and is completely surrounded by an inflammation that is so severe that it brings about fever and great danger. One should put a strong, caustic remedy on the burned site and a cataplasm on the surrounding inflammation. This cataplasm should combine [medications] that repel and prevent the surrounding inflammation from spreading and that have a cooling and dissolving effect on it. *Qāṭājānas* 5.[2]

رب يسر

المقالة الخامسة عشر

تشتمل على فصول تتعلق بأعمال اليد

١. القروح العفنة التي تنتشر وتسعى إلى ما حولها تحتاج إلى أدوية قوية جدا.
ومرارا شتّى يحتاج في علاجها إلى استعمال الكيّ بالنار. خامسة قاطاجانس.

٢. من القروح قروح يقال لها الجمرة وهي قرحة تحدث في موضعها شبيهة
بحرق النار وورم شديد يستدير حول الموضع كلّه ويبلغ من شدّة الورم أن يجلب
الحمّى وأخطار عظيمة. وينبغي أن يجعل على موضع حرق النار دواء قوي من الأدوية
الكاوية ويجعل على الورم الذي حولها ضماد يجمع ردع ومنع ما يتحلّب وتطفئة وتحليل
لما في الورم. خامسة قاطاجانس.

---

١ بسم الله الرحمن الرحيم رب يسر] om. ELBOU ‖ ٣ الخامسة] لحبيش ‖ add. U
٩ حرق النار] الحرق ELBOU

(3) One should not cauterize a part of the body that has depth or hollowness—all bodily parts have depth or hollowness except the hands, feet, and loins. *In Hippocratis De aeris [aquis locis] commentarius* 2.[3]

(4) If pus has collected in the area between the chest and the lungs and one despairs of cleansing it through expectoration, apply cauterization to the chest. *In Hippocratis Aphorismos commentarius* 6.[4]

(5) Says Moses: Consider how he recommends doing so only in the case of despair. Therefore, it does not contradict his previous statement in [his commentary] on *De aeris [aquis locis]* 2.

(6) Cauterization with a glowing hot iron or with caustic remedies should be applied to those sites that are affected by a severe illness caused by a surplus of humors or by their bad quality, as in the case of malignant ulcers. *In Hippocratis Epidemiarum* 6.6.[5]

(7) One should not hasten to puncture the abdomen of a dropsy patient. One is forced to do so only when so much moisture collects in it that it bears heavily upon the patient and weakens him. One should hasten to cauterize the chest of patients with lung ulcers before they are eaten away by corrosion. *In Hippocratis Epidemiarum* 6.7.[6]

(8) If you lance a site and evacuate the pus from it, be careful at that moment and thereafter not to use oil or water [to wash the wound]. When you have to wash the wound, do so with hydromel, or vinegar mixed [with water], or wine alone, or wine mixed with honey. *Ad Glauconem [de methodo medendi]* 2.[7]

٣. لا ينبغي أن يكوى عضوله غور أو بطن وليس في البدن عضو إلا وله بطن أو غور خلا اليدين والرجلين والحقوين. في شرحه للثانية من الأهوية.

٤. إذا كانت المذة قد اجتمع منها فيما بين الصدر والرئة ما يؤيس من استقائه بالنفث فاستعمل الكيّ على الصدر. في شرحه لسادسة الفصول.

٥. قال موسى: تأمّل كيف لم يأمر بهذا إلا عند اليأس. ولذلك لا يناقض هذا ما تقدّم له ذكره في ثانية الأهوية.

٦. الكيّ بالحديد المحمّى أو بالأدوية المحرقة ينبغي أن يستعمل في المواضع التي ينزل بها من العلل أمر عظيم من كثرة الأخلاط و رداءتها كالذي يكون في القروح الخبيثة. في السادسة من شرحه لسادسة أبيديميا.

٧. ليس ينبغي أن يبادر في ثقب بطن المستسقي وإنما يضطرّ إليه إذا كثرت الرطوبة حتى تثقل المريض وتوهنه. وينبغي أن يبادر بكيّ صدور أصحاب قرحة الرئة قبل أن تتأكّل القرحة. في السابعة من شرحه لسادسة أبيديميا.

٨. إذا بطّطت موضعا واستفرغت ما فيه من المذة فاحذر في ذلك الوقت وفيما بعده أن تستعمل الدهن أو الماء. ومتى احتجت أن تغسل الجرح فإنما ينبغي لك أن تغسله بماء العسل أو الخلّ الممزوج أو الشراب أو الشراب وحده أو الشراب المخلوط بالعسل. ثانية أغلوقن.

١ لا ينبغي...والحقوين] ومنع أيضا من الكيّ للأعضاء التي لها غور سيّما إذا كان للعضو بطن غائر فإنّ للأعضاء كلّها بطونا ما خلا اليدين والرجلين والفخذين fol. 73r C | بطن] باطن L | بطن] باطن L || ٣ المذة] المادة ELBO | فيما] om. ELBO || ٩ أبيديميا] أفيديميا ELOU || ١٠ ينبغي أن] G¹ || ١٢ أبيديميا] أفيديميا ELOU || ١٣ واستفرغت] واستخرجت ELOU || ١٥ أو الشراب وحده] om. EL

(9) Malignant ulcers that putrefy need medications that are so extremely sharp that they are similar to fire, such as vitriol, yellow vitriol, the two types of arsenic, and lime. For the burning of these medications is like the burning of fire; and often we use fire in [treat-
5   ing] these kinds of ulcers when these medications are overpowered and cannot have any effect on them. But sometimes these medications are beneficial for the disease called carbuncles when they are put on the site of the eschar, because this is the site that putrefies [more than any other].[8] They should not be applied to the surrounding area. *Ad Glauconem [de
10   methodo medendi]* 2.[9]

(10) When a limb dies to the point that one does not feel it when it is pricked, cut off, or burned with fire and inevitably turns black, hasten to cut it off at the point where it touches the connected healthy site. *Ad Glauconem [de methodo medendi]* 2.[10]

15   (11) Medications which are beneficial for putrid sites are bitter vetch [*Vicia ervilia* Willd] with vinegar, darnel [*Lolium temulentum*] flour with honey,[11] bean flour with oxymel, a dried pastille, or bean [*Vicia faba*] flour with oxymel and salt. Select from these and the like according to the temperament of the patient. *Ad Glauconem [de methodo medendi]* 2.[12]

20   (12) When you amputate a limb that has putrefied or died, be careful and cautious and use those medications that I have described, after examining the nature of the patient and the nature of the limb. Once you have amputated the limb, cauterize its root, as we often do in the case of pudenda.[13] *Ad Glauconem [de methodo medendi]* 2.[14]

25   (13) I [have] treated the illness of cancer at its beginning many times, and it was cured. However, if the illness becomes serious and the tumor greatly enlarged, nobody is capable of curing it except through surgery, in order to excise the tumor and completely uproot it all around until one reaches a healthy spot. But if there are large vessels—especially

٩. القروح الخبيثة التي تكون معها عفونة تحتاج من الأدوية إلى ما هو منها

في غاية الحدّة حتّى يضارع قوّته قوّة النار مثل الزاج والقلقطار والزرنيخين والنورة.

فقد تحرق هذه الأدوية كما تحرق النار وكثيرا ما نستعمل النار في مثل هذه القروح

إذا غلبت هذه الأدوية واستعصت عن فعلها فيها. وقد تصلح هذه الأدوية للعلّة

المعروفة بالجمرة إذا وضعت على موضع الخشكريشة لأنّ هذا الموضع هو الذي نالته

العفونة ولا ينبغي أن يوضع على ما حوله. ثانية أغلوقن.

١٠. العضو إذا مات حتّى لا يحسّ إذا أنت نخسته أو قطعته أو أحرقته بالنار

وهو بلا محالة يسودّ فينبغي أن تبادر إلى قطعه من حيث يلقى الموضع الصحيح الذي يتّصل

به. ثانية أغلوقن.

١١. الأدوية التي تصلح للمواضع التي تعفن الكرسنة بالخلّ ودقيق الشيلم بالعسل

ودقيق الباقلّى والخلّ والعسل أو بعض الأقراص المجفّفة أو دقيق الباقلّى وخلّ وعسل

وملح. يختار من هذه وما أشبهها بحسب مزاج الشخص. ثانية أغلوقن.

١٢. إذا قطعت عضوا قد عفن أو قد مات فخذ بالوثيقة والتحرّز واستعمل

الأدوية التي وصفتها بعد أن تنظر في طبيعة من تعالجه وطبيعة العضو. فإذا قطعت

العضو تكوي أصله كما نفعل كثيرا في الفروج. ثانية أغلوقن.

١٣. السرطان هذه العلّة في الابتداء قد عالجناها مرارا كثيرة فبرأت. فأمّا إذا

تفاقم الأمر وعظم الورم عظما ذا قدر فما أحد وصل إلى التأتّي لبرء ها إلا بعلاج

الحديد ليقطع الورم ويستأصل الورم بأسره كما يدور حتّى يبلغ الموضع الصحيح. إلا

---

٤ فيها] om. G || ٩ ثانية أغلوقن] في مقالته تلك ELO || ١٢ ثانية أغلوقن] في مقالته تلك

ELO || ١٥ تكوي] تداوي L | في الفروج] om. B : في القروح E(?)GLOU | ثانية

أغلوقن] في مقالته تلك ELO

pulsatile—one cannot be sure but that it may start to bleed immediately; and if the tumor is also close to a vital organ, excision is dangerous, because it is impossible to cauterize the root of the disease because of its proximity to a vital organ. *Ad Glauconem [de methodo medendi]* 2.[15]

(14) Those suffering from dizziness and vertigo or various types of severe headache, such as migraine or a headache affecting the whole head,[16] sometimes benefit from venesection of the pulsatile vessels behind the ear. But sometimes they do not benefit from it because the vapors that produce these illnesses rise to the brain through other pulsatile vessels that are not visible on the surface of the body and that ascend to the cerebral plexus. *De locis affectis* 3.[17]

(15) Someone suffering from any wound at any site of the body—a site that has tendons and nerves and is free from flesh and has many bones—is in danger and on the verge of being afflicted by pain, sleeplessness, spasms, and delirium. *De methodo [medendi]* 4.[18]

(16) When a part of the body is sensitive, treat it with a medication that causes minimal pain. But you may treat a part that has little sensitivity with very strong drugs, when the disease requires a strong kind of treatment. *De methodo [medendi]* 4.[19]

(17) If someone is pricked [directly] in a nerve and he suffers unavoidably, because of the great sensitivity of the nerve, from severe pain, exercise your skill to alleviate the pain and to prevent inflammation [of the site]. This [should be done] by keeping the site open and by not allowing it to heal up, and by, as a precautionary measure, increasing the tear in the skin.[20] Phlebotomize [the patient] if he is strong enough to tolerate it; and, when his body contains bad humors, evacuate them by [giving him] a purgative. Foment the site where he is pricked with extremely thin olive oil—that is, old and heated. Be extremely careful not to do so with hot water, because this putrefies the nerve and the patient will die. *De methodo [medendi]* 6.[21]

أنه إن كان عروق غلاظ ولا سيّما ضاربة فليس يؤمن النزف على المكان وإن كان الورم أيضا بالقرب من عضو نفيس فإنّ قطعه خطرا إذ لا يمكن أن يكوى أصل العلّة لقربه من عضو نفيس . ثانية أغلوقن.

١٤. أصحاب الدوار والسدر وأنواع الصداع الشديد كالشقيقة والخوذة قد ينتفعون بقطع العروق الضاربة التي خلف الأذنين. وقد لا ينتفعون بذلك لأن تكون تلك الأبخرة المولّدة لتلك الأمراض تصعد إلى الدماغ في عروق أُخَر ضوارب غير ظاهرة في سطح الجسم وترقى إلى شبكة الدماغ. ثالثة التعرّف.

١٥. كلّ جراحة تكون في أيّ موضع كان من البدن وذلك الموضع ذو أوتار وأعصاب أو معرق معرّى من اللحم كثير العظام فإن صاحبها على خطر وشرف من أن يعرض له وجع وسهر وتشنّج واختلاط عقل. رابعة الحيلة.

١٦. ما كان من الأعضاء حسّاسا فينبغي لك أن تعالجه علاجا في غاية البعد عن أن يوجع ويؤلِم. وما كان من الأعضاء عسر الحسّ فقد يمكّنك أن تعالجه بأدوية معها فضل قوة إن احتاج المرض لذلك العلاج القوي. رابعة الحيلة.

١٧. إذا أصابت عصبة من العصب نخسة فلا بدّ له ضرورة لفضل حسّ العصب من الوجع الشديد فاحتل في تسكين الوجع ومنع حدوث الورم. وذلك بأن تبقي الموضع مفتوحا لا تلحمه ومن الحزم أن تزيد في خرق الجلد. وتقصد إن كانت القوة محتملة وإن كان رديء الأخلاط فنستفرغ الخلط الرديء بالدواء المسهل. ينطل موضع النخسة بزيت في غاية اللطافة أعني عتيق مسخّن. واحذر كل الحذر أن تقربه بماء حارّ لأنه يعفن العصب ويهلك العليل. سادسة الحيلة.

---

٢ نفيس فإن قطعه خطرا إذ لا يمكن أن يكوى أصل العلّة لقربه من عضو] om. B | فإنّ] فإن] كان

ELOU | والخوذة...متى (XV، ٥٠)] om. O | ٧ إلى شبكة] لشبكة ELBU ||

٨ تكون في أيّ موضع كان] في أيّ موضع كانت EL : في أيّ موضع كان U | ١٥ فاحتل]

فاحتال ELBU | ١٦ لا تلحمه] ملحما L

(18) If you choose to treat a cancer through surgery, begin by evacuating the melancholic humor through purgation. Then excise the entire site until not even the root thereof remains. Let the blood flow, and do not hasten to stop it. Then compress the surrounding vessels and press the thick blood out of them. Treat [it in the same way as other] ulcers.[22] *De methodo [medendi]* 14.[23]

(19) Scrofula is a hard tumor that arises in the soft flesh.[24] If it arises in the soft flesh that was created for an important function—namely, that which was created for the production of the sputum and the like— and pulsatile and nonpulsatile vessels are connected to it, its therapy should be similar to that of other hard tumors. But [the scrofula] arising in the soft flesh created to fill up empty space and to support the vessels should be treated through extirpation of the bad organ in its entirety. This [can be done] either through surgery, as is done in the case of cancer, or by letting it putrefy. *De methodo [medendi]* 14.[25]

(20) The therapy of abscesses which mostly occur on the surface of the body has three common goals: dissolution, putrefaction, or surgery. For honeylike[26] [abscesses], one needs only one of these [forms of therapy]. Those [abscesses] whose contents resemble meal boiled in water[27] may be either excised or allowed to putrefy. Fatlike [abscesses][28] can only be treated through surgery, since they cannot putrefy nor dissolve. *De methodo [medendi]* 14.[29]

(21) Excess flesh in the inner angle of the eye[30] and excrescences on the anus—namely, hemorrhoids—require surgery. *De methodo [medendi]* 14.[31]

(22) If you consider applying surgery to any part of the body, strive for three things: the first is to complete your work in the shortest time possible; the second is that no pain at all should be felt during the surgery; and the third is the question of safety. This latter goal is achieved by observing three things: the first is that you are sure that your goal

١٨. إن أنت اخترت أن تعالج السرطان بالحديد فاجعل مبدأك استفراغ الخلط السوداوي بالإسهال. ثمّ اقطع على موضع العلّة كلّه حتّى لا يبق لها أصل بتّة. ودع الدم يسيل ولا تعجل في حبسه واغمزعلى ما حوله من العروق واعصرمنها الدم الغليظ. ثمّ داوي القرحة. أخيرة الحيلة.

١٩. الخنازيرهي و رم صلب يحدث في اللحم الرخو. فإن حدث هذا في اللحم الرخو المخلوق لمنفعة عظيمة وهو الذي خلق لتوليد الريق ونحوه وتتّصل به عروق ضوارب وغير ضوارب فإنّ مداواته كمداواة سائرالأورام الصلبة. فأمّا الحادث في اللحم الرخو المخلوق لحشو الفرج وإدعام العروق فقد يداوى بقلع العضوالردي ء بجملته وذلك إمّا بقطعه بالحديدكما يفعل بالسرطان وإمّا بتعفينه. أخيرة الحيلة.

٢٠. الدبيلات الأكثرية الحدوث في سطح الجسم الأغراض العاميّة في مداواتها ثلاثة: التحليل أوالتعفين أوالقطع بالحديد. فالعسلية منها تحتاج إلى إحدى هذه فقط. وأمّا التي تكون الذي داخلها كالدقيق المطبوخ بالماء فيجوز أن تقطعها ويجوز أن تعفنها. وأمّا الشحمية فإنّها تعالج بالحديد فقط إذ كانت لا يمكن فيها أن تعفن ولا أن تتحلّل. أخيرة الحيلة.

٢١. اللحم الزائد في مأق العين والزوائد النابتة في المقعدة وهي البواسير تحتاج أن تقطع. أخيرة الحيلة.

٢٢. إذا هممت بقطع شيء من الجسم بالحديد فاقصد ثلاثة أغراض: أحدها أن يكون فعلك يتمّ في أقصرما يمكن من الزمان والثاني أن لا يكون هناك وجع بوجه عند ما تقطع أمرالعافية والثالث أمرالعافية. وأمرالعافية يكون بثلاثة أغراض: أوّلها أن تتيقّن

---

٢ اقطع] G¹ || ٧ وغير ضوارب] om. EL || ٨ بقلع] بقطع ELU || ١٢ الذي] ما في EL : التي B || ١٤ أخيرة الحيلة] في مقالله تلك EL || ١٥ اللحم...الحيلة] om. B | مأق] أماق L || ١٧ إذا] ما add. LU | الجسم] الجسم G : الشحم] الشحم B | الجنس B || ١٩ والثالث] G¹

can be absolutely realized;[32] the second is that, if your goal is not realized, [the patient] will not come to any harm because of that;[33] and the third is that you are sure that the disease will not return. If you observe these three goals, it will be evident to you that sometimes surgery is preferable, but at other times the application of medications [is preferable]. *De methodo [medendi]* 14.[34]

(23) If vessels in the legs or testicles become thick,[35] they should be excised and extirpated. Similarly, an excrescence in the nose[36] should be excised, together with the covering internal membrane, and, in some cases, together with the entire nose.[37] *De methodo [medendi]* 14.[38]

(24) As long as the pterygium[39] in the eye is small, it can be treated with cleansing medications similar to medications for trachoma. If it increases and hardens, it should be treated by surgery. *De methodo [medendi]* 14.[40]

(25) Hailstone in the eyelid [chalazion][41] requires excision. The same applies to the pus collected in the eye in the illness called *kumna*.[42] However, in most cases it can be treated with dissolving medications that do not have a strong drying effect, because these evacuate most of the pus and congeal the rest. I have evacuated this pus by lancing the hornlike tunic in the rim. It can also be evacuated by shaking the head until the pus descends. *De methodo [medendi]* 14.[43]

(26) For the treatment of illnesses associated with pain,[44] one should, first of all, use those medicines which are moist and slightly heating. Then [use] slackening medicines, namely, those which loosen the stretching of the organs. *Qāṭājānas* 7.[45]

(27) The uvula can be affected by the illness of extreme relaxation without an inflammation, in which case we generally cut it off. But when the uvula is affected by this illness, remedies that heat and that

أنّ غرضك يتمّ ضرورة والثاني أنّه إذا لم يتمّ غرضك لا ينال بسبب ذلك مضرّة والثالث أن تثق بأنّ المرض لا يعود. فإذا نظرت في هذه الثلاثة الأغراض يتبيّن لك أنّ في بعض علاج الحديد أفضل وفي بعض الأوقات استعمال الأدوية أفضل. أخيرة الحيلة.

٢٣. إذا غلظت عروق في الساقين والخصيتين فإنها تقطع وتستأصل. وكذلك اللحم الزائد في الأنف يقطع مع الطبقة الملبّسة من داخل وقد يقطع مع الأنف بجملته. أخيرة الحيلة.

٢٤. مداواة الظفرة التي تكون في العين ما دامت صغيرة بالأدوية التي تجلو بمنزلة أدوية الجرب. وإذا تزيّدت وصلبت تداوى بالحديد. أخيرة الحيلة.

٢٥. البردة تحتاج إلى قطع. وكذلك القيح المجتمع في العين في العلّة التي يقال لها الكمنة أكثر ما تداوى بأدوية تحلّل لا بما يجفّف تجفيفا قويا لأنّه يستفرغ معظمها ويحمد البقية. وقد استفرغنا نحن هذا القيح بأن بطّنا الطبقة القرنية في موضع الإكليل. ويستفرغ أيضا بهزّ الرأس حتّى ينزل القيح إلى أسفل. أخيرة الحيلة.

٢٦. أوّل ما ينبغي أن يستعمل من الأدوية في علاج الأدواء التي معها وجع ما كان منها رطبا وكان مع ذلك يسخّن قليلا. ثمّ الأدوية المرخية وهي التي تحلّ تمديد الأعضاء. سابعة قاطاجانس.

٢٧. تحدث علّة في اللهاة أن تسترخي استرخاء شديدا من غير ورم وقد جرت عادتنا حينئذ أن نقطعها. وبالحقيقة أنّ اللهاة إذا كانت بها هذه العلّة فإنّ الأدوية

---

٣ علاج الحديد أفضل وفي بعض الأوقات] G^1 || ٧ أخيرة الحيلة] في مقالبه تلك EL ||
٩ أخيرة الحيلة] في مقالبه تلك EL || ١٠ البردة] الطرفة L || ١٢ البقية] البقي L ||
١٣ بهزّ] om. L : به B | أخيرة الحيلة] في مقالبه تلك EL || ١٤ في علاج] لعلاج E :
ليعالج L || ١٦ سابعة] رابعة EL || ١٧ تحدث] قد تحدث L

cleanse the phlegm are really beneficial for it, because, at that time, the uvula mostly tends to turn white, as if it were lacking blood. *Mayāmir* 6.[46]

(28) The eye is the most sensitive of organs. Therefore, drip medications into it after extremely gently lifting the upper eyelid. The medications should be steeped in a liquid that does not bite. The ancient [physicians] were very much in the right to use egg white [as a base for eyedrops]. *De methodo [medendi]* 13.[47]

(29) A moist, liquid medicine stays at its place only when applied in a ligament. Therefore, medicines for lachrymal fistula should be dry, because the ligament has to cover the whole eye, and the eye cannot tolerate being constantly bandaged for so many days that the fistula in it is cured. *Mayāmir* 5.[48]

(30) When [in the case of a cataract operation] the moisture has descended from the surface of the pupil, the couching needle[49] should be held for a long time in the place [where] one wants the moisture to settle, so that it becomes firmly fixed there. *De officina [medici]* 1.[50]

(31) If you dissect the hornlike tunic, the first thing you find is a fine and thin liquid streaming and pouring out. It is the moisture that you often see flowing out from the opening made in the eye that is being operated [on] for a cataract. This is followed by the whole eye becoming shriveled, contracted, and hollow. *De usu [partium]* 10.[51]

(32) The most beneficial and appropriate medication for nerve wounds is that which dries while it is slightly warming, or one in which the heat is not noticeable but which dries just the same. Everything that has the property to attract moistures from the depth of the body to the outside is suitable for nerve wounds. *Qāṭājānas* 6.[52]

التي تُسخن وتنقّي البلغم نافعة لها وهي تكون في ذلك الوقت على الأمر الأكثر مائلة إلى البياض وكأنها عديمة الدم. سادسة الميامر.

٢٨. العين أكثر الأعضاء حسًّا ولهذا ينبغي أن تقطر الأدوية فيها بعد أن يترفّق برفع الجفن الأعلى على غاية الرفق. وتذيف الأدوية برطوبة طبيعتها بعيدة عن التلذيع.

٥ وقد أصاب القدماء في بياض البيض جدًّا. ثالثة عشر الحيلة.

٢٩. الدواء الرطب السيّال لا يلبث إلا برباط ولذلك تجعل أدوية الغرب يابسة لأنّ الرباط يحتاج أن يكون على العين كلّها. والعين لا تحتمل أن تربط برباط لا يفارقها أيّامًا كثيرة بمقدار يبرأ فيه الناصور. خامسة الميامر.

٣٠. الماء من بعد ما ينزل ويخطّ عن وجه الناظر ينبغي أن يمسك بالمقدح مدّة

١٠ طويلة في المواضع التي يراد أن يستقرّ فيها كي يتشبّث بها. في الأولى من الحانوت.

٣١. إذا شققت الصفاق القرني كان أوّل ما تلقاه الرطوبة اللطيفة الرقيقة فتنصبّ وتسيل وهي الرطوبة التي كثيرًا ما تراها تسيل وتخرج من الثقب الذي ينثقب في العين التي يقدح منها الماء. ثمّ يتلو ذلك تَشنّج العين بأسرها وتقلّصها وغورانها. عاسرة المنافع.

٣٢. أنفع الأدوية لجراحات العصب وأصلحها له ما كان يجفّف وهو يسير

١٥ الحرارة أو تكون حرارته خافية ويجفّف مع ذلك. وكلّ ما شأنه أن يجذب الرطوبات من عمق البدن إلى ظاهره يوافق جراحات العصب. ثالثة قاطاجانس.

٤ عن] من EL || ٦ الغرب] الجرب EL || ٩ الماء...يتشبّث بها] الماء من بعد ما ينزل ويخطّ عن وجه الناظر ينبغي أن يمسك بالمقدح مدّة طويلة في المواضع التي يراد أن يستفرغ فيها ويتثبّت بها تثبّتا وثيقا °Alī ibn Riḍwān, *Compendium of Galen's commentary on Hippocrates'* *KAT' IHTREION*, ed. Lyons, p. 104, l. 12 || ١٠ يراد] يكاد L || ١١ كان] فإن L || ١١ له] به EL

(33) As medications for nerve wounds, I use sulphur that has not been affected by fire, [mixed] with olive oil until it assumes the consistency of bath sordes.[53] Sometimes, for young people and those of similar constitution, I use mastic from the turpentine tree [*Pistacia terebinthus*] alone, or with spurge [*Euphorbia resinifera* Berg. and var.] for dry bodies. Similarly, I use bee glue[54] alone or with spurge kneaded with old olive oil. For very hard bodies, I use sagapenum, sometimes with old olive oil and sometimes with mastic from the turpentine tree—so, too, opopanax.[55] Sometimes I also mix the olive oil with washed lime. *De methodo [medendi]* 6.[56]

(34) If a nerve lies bare and exposed by the wound, use none of the aforementioned strong medications, but use only lime that has been washed very well with thin olive oil; heat this, and then apply it. *De methodo [medendi]* 6.[57]

(35) If any organ is affected by a large tumor, it is dangerous to evacuate the pus therefrom all at once, because the patient will immediately suffer from syncope and from a collapse of his strength. This is because the pus obstructs, as it were, the openings of the pulsatile vessels; and if the entire pus is evacuated [all at once], a large amount of pneuma is expelled all at once. *In Hippocratis Aphorismos commentarius* 6.[58]

(36) The evacuation of water retained in the abdomen of someone suffering from ascites is effected either through dissolving drugs or through puncturing the peritoneum by surgery. But the fluid collected in the scrotum[59] should be evacuated by a tube inserted into it. Sometimes, a part of the membrane [containing the fluid] should be excised in the case of hydrocele. Similarly, the uvula should be excised in some cases [with the disease itself].[60] Do not hurry to excise it, [but wait] until much time has passed and it has turned as thin as a thong;[61] then excise it. *De methodo [medendi]* 14.[62]

(37) In abdominal wounds, always take care that the side of the wound is higher than the other side. If the wound is on the right side, turn the patient on his left side; and if the wound is on the left side,

٣٣. أمّا أدوية جراحات العصب فإنّي أستعمل فيها الكبريت الذي لم تصبها النار مع الزيت حتّى يصير في ثخانة وسخ الحمّام. وقد أستعمل في أبدان الصبيان ونحوهم علك البطم وحده أو مع الفربيون في الأبدان الجافة. وكذلك أستعمل وسخ الكور وحده أو مع الفربيون معجون بزيت عتيق. وأمّا الأبدان الشديدة الصلابة فأستعمل فيها السكبينج مرّة مع زيت عتيق ومرّة مع علك البطم وكذلك الجاوشير. وقد أخلط مع الزيت أيضا نورة مغسولة. سادسة الحيلة.

٣٤. متى كانت العصبة ظاهرة مكشوفة في الجراحة فلا تقاربها بشيء من الأدوية القوية المتقدّم ذكرها ويكفيك نورة مغسولة جدّا بزيت لطيف، تسخن الدواء وحينئذ تضعه. سادسة الحيلة.

٣٥. إذا حدث في أحد من الأعضاء ورم عظيم فاستفراغ القيح منه دفعة واحدة خطر لأنّه يحدث لصاحبه على المكان الغشي وسقوط القوة لأنّ المدّة كأنّها سدّ في فوهات العروق الضوارب. وإذا استفرغت المدّة كلّها خرج معها شيء كثير من الروح دفعة. في شرحه لسادسة الفصول.

٣٦. استفراغ الماء المحتقن في بطن من به الاستسقاء الزقّي يكون إمّا بأدوية محلّلة وإمّا بثقب الصفاق بالحديد. وأمّا الرطوبة المجتمعة في قيلة الماء فتستفرغ بأنبوب يدخل فيها. وقد يقطع في القيلة جزء من الصفاق وكذلك اللهاة تقطع. ولا تعجل في قطعها حتّى يطول بها الزمان وترقّ كالسير وحينئذ تقطع. أخيرة الحيلة.

٣٧. اجعل قصدك دائما في جراحات البطن أن تجعل الناحية التي فيها الجراحة أرفع من الناحية الأخرى. إن كانت الجراحة في الشقّ الأيمن فتميل العليل على الشقّ

---

turn him on the right side. After suturing the wound, apply bandages as necessary. *De methodo [medendi]* 6.[63]

(38) For any fresh ulcer, except abdominal ones, it is appropriate that blood exude from the wound itself, whether little or much; for, if blood flows therefrom, the ulcer and the surrounding area will be less inflamed. *De methodo [medendi]* 4.[64]

(39) When an excessive amount of blood is streaming from wounds because the vessels have burst, the flow of the blood can be stopped either by cauterization, or by drugs whose strength is equal to cautery, or by something that closes and agglutinates, or by transferring it to a nearby site,[65] or by attracting it to the opposite side, or by cooling the whole body and especially the part of the body where the wound is. Many times, [the bleeding] is stopped by drinking cold water, or by the external application of vinegar mixed [with water],[66] of astringent acidic wine, or of other substances with cooling and astringent properties. *De methodo [medendi]* 5.[67]

(40) If the hemorrhage is from a pulsatile vessel, the bleeding can be stopped by one of two things: either by tying a ligature around it; or by cutting and severing it into two halves, so that each part shrinks and contracts to the nearby side and becomes covered with flesh. Sometimes we are forced to do the same for a nonpulsatile vessel, if the vessel is large or if it is situated in a major part where there is great danger. The most prudent practice is to do both things simultaneously, applying a ligature to the root of the vessel close to the heart or liver and cutting it into two halves. *De methodo [medendi]* 5.[68]

(41) We are forced to cauterize if the hemorrhage is caused by corrosion or putrefaction affecting it. Similarly, if we cut off a part because of corrosion or putrefaction that crept into it, we cauterize its root or apply caustic astringent drugs to it, such as vitriol and the like. *De methodo [medendi]* 5.[69]

(42) In the case of old ulcers, blood should flow from [the ulcer], either much or little. If the diseased part has turned livid[70] or black or red, we scarify it, let it bleed, and place a dry sponge on it. Then we

الأيسر وإن كانت في الأيسر مال على الأيمن. بعد خياطة الجراحة ولفّها على ما ينبغي. سادسة الحيلة.

٣٨. كلّ قرحة طريئة أية قرحة كانت غير القرحة التي تكون في البطن فينبغي أن يخرج من الجرح نفسه دم إمّا قليل أوكثير فإنه إذا جرى منه الدم كان تورّم القرحة وتورّم ما حولها أقلّ. رابعة الحيلة.

٣٩. الجراحات التي يفرط خروج الدم منها لانبثاق العروق فقد يقطع ذلك الدم بالكيّ أو بأدوية قوتها قوة الكيّ أو بما يسدّ ويلصق أو بنقله إلى قرب المواضع أو بجذبه إلى خلاف الجهة أو بتبريد جملة البدن وبخاصّة بتبريد العضو الذي فيه الجرح. وكثيرا ما ينقطع بشربه ماء بارد وبالخلّ الممزوج وبالشراب القابض العفص وسائر ما شأنه أن يبرّد ويقبض إذا صبّ من خارج. خامسة الحيلة.

٤٠. إن كان العرق المنبثق منه الدم عرق ضاربا فإنّ الدم ينقطع بأحد أمرين: إمّا بأن يستوثق منه برباط وإمّا بقطعه قطعا يبتره بنصفين كي يتقلّص كلّ قسم ويتكمّش إلى الجانب الذي يليه ويتغطّى باللحم. وقد يضطرّتا الأمر إلى هذا العمل في عرق غير ضارب إذا كان عرقا عظيما أو في عضو شريف جليل الخطر. والأحزم أن تعمل الأمرين جميعا فتربط أصل العرق ممّا يلي القلب أو الكبد وتقطعه بنصفين. خامسة الحيلة.

٤١. يضطرّتا الأمر إلى الكيّ إذا كان انبعاث الدم بسبب أكلة وقعت في عضو أو بسبب عفونة أصابته. وكذلك إذا قطعنا عضوا من أجل أكلة أو عفونة دبّت فيه فإنّا نكوي أصله بالنار أو بأدوية محرقة قابضة كالزاج وأنواعه. خامسة الحيلة.

٤٢. القروح العتيقة ينبغي أن يخرج منها دم إمّا كثير وإمّا قليل. وإن كان العضو العليل قد اخضرّ أو اسودّ أو احمرّ شرطناه وأخرجنا دمه و وضعنا عليه

٣ أيّة] أيّ EL | غير [om. ELBU || ٦ لانبثاق [L²: لاختناق LU || ٧ ويلصق ويلزق ELBU

treat it with medicines that have a drying effect. If it is necessary to bleed it a second time, we do so again. *De methodo [medendi]* 4.[71]

(43) If you see that only the rim of an ulcer has changed in color or become hard, you should cut it out and uproot it until [you reach] healthy flesh. If that change has spread over a large area, you should either uproot it or treat it with medicines for a long time. *De methodo [medendi]* 4.[72]

(44) If some pus has usually streamed from a fistula for a long time but then the flow is stopped, one should open [the blockage]. *In Hippocratis Epidemiarum* 6.2.[73]

(45) Sometimes, a sinuous ulcer,[74] when it is very dirty, can be syringed with lye from ashes,[75] which is called *al-qāṭir*,[76] or with hydromel. The less dirty it is, the less honey should be used. Hereafter, one may also syringe [the sinuous ulcer] with wine mixed with honey. Hydromel is more effective for cleansing [the pus from the sinuous ulcer], while wine is more beneficial for promoting adhesion after the cleansing. Then put a plaster with agglutinant drugs on it, put a new sponge steeped in wine thereon, and bind [these] onto it. Begin tying it from the bottom of the sinuous ulcer and end at its opening, so that it presses on the ulcer without causing pain. Change the bandage once every three days. Put on [another] small cloth, [applying it] in a circular form,[77] with a plaster on the opening of the ulcer. When the bottom of the sinuous ulcer extends downward and the opening upward, and you cannot change this [position], make an incision in the bottom part, so that its contents may flow out. *Ad Glauconem [de methodo medendi]* 2.[78]

(46) When there is a severe hemorrhage from a pulsatile or nonpulsatile vessel, we concern ourselves with the vessel and cut it transversely, because, although it never closes up,[79] we will rescue the patient from the danger [he is in]. Similarly, if a nerve is affected by an accident or puncture, we are often forced to cut it transversely and to abolish a movement in order to save the patient from the danger of [being afflicted] by spasms or delirium or both. Similarly, when a major joint

إسفنجة يابسة ثمّ نداويه بأدوية تجفّف. وإن احتاج إلى معاودة استفراغ الدم منه استفرغناه ثانية. رابعة الحيلة.

٤٣. متى رأيت شقّة القرحة قد تغيّر لونها وحدها أو وصلت فينبغي أن تقطع وتستأصل إلى اللحم الصحيح. وإن كان ذلك التغيّر قد أمعن إلى مسافة كثيرة فإمّا أن تستأصله أو تداويه بالأدوية في مدّة طويلة. رابعة الحيلة.

٤٤. إذا كان الناصور قد جرت العادة مدّة طويلة أن يسيل منه شيء، ثمّ احتقن ما كان يسيل منه فينبغي أن تفتحه. في الثانية من شرحه لسادسة أبيديميا.

٤٥. قد يحقن المخبأ إذا كان وضرا جدًا بماء الرماد وهو الذي يسمّى القاطر أو بماء وعسل. وكلّما كان أقلّ وضرا قلّل العسل ويحقن أيضا بعد ذلك بالشراب الممزوج بالعسل. وماء العسل في التنقية أبلغ والشراب على الإلزاق الكائن بعد التنقية أعون. وضع المرهم الذي شأنه أن يلصق من فوق واجعل على المرهم إسفنجا جديدا مبلولا بشراب وقطّ من فوقه وابتدئ من الشدّ من أسفل المخبأ وانته إلى فمه حتّى يضغطه من غير أن يؤلمه وحلّه كلّ ثلاثة أيّام مرّة. واجعل على ضمام يطبق. وإن كان أسفل المخبأ أسفل وفمه فوق ولا تقدر على تغيّر وضعه فشقّه من أسفل كي يسيل ما فيه. ثانية أغلوقن.

٤٦. متى انبثق دم مفرط من عرق ضارب أو غير ضارب فإنّا نعمد إلى العرق ونبتره عرضا وإن كان ذلك لا يلتئم أبدا، لكن نخلّص صاحب العلّة من الخطر. وكذلك متى أصابت عصبة وجبة أو نخسة فيضطرّنا ذلك كم مرّة أن نبترها عرضا ونبطل حركة من الحركات لنخلّص صاحب العلّة من التشنّج أو اختلاط العقل أو كليهما. وعلى هذا

١ احتاج] احتجنا L ‖ ٧ أبيديميا] ELBU ‖ الحيلة G: أفديميا ‖ ١١ يلصق] يلزق ELBU ‖ جديدا] غير L ‖ ١٤ تغيّر] G¹ ‖ ١٦ متى انبثق] من انبثق منه G ‖ ١٨ أصابت عصبة] أصاب عصبه G

suffers from a dislocation in combination with an ulcer, we treat the ulcer [first] until it is healed, even if it is not possible to treat the dislocation afterwards. For if we try to combine the reduction of the dislocation with the treatment of the ulcer, the [patient] is usually affected by

5   spasms. Therefore, we should treat the more dangerous [condition first]. *De methodo [medendi]* 3.[80]

(47) The following medicine stops a hemorrhage, even from the jugular veins:[81] Take frankincense [gum resin of *Boswellia Carterii* and var.], or pulverized frankincense and aloe, and mix these with egg white until

10   the medicine assumes the consistency of honey. Smear this upon the hairs of a hare, and apply it to the torn vessel and the entire wound, and bandage it well. But beware of [causing pain], because there is nothing in the world that is more effective in provoking a hemorrhage than pain. Then loosen the bandage after three days; and if you find

15   the medicine still firmly adherent to the wound, do not remove it, but put [more] of the same medicine thereon, moistening, as it were, the hairs of the hare. Then bandage it in the same way as the first [time that you bandaged it]. If the hairs of the hare fall off, replace them and apply the bandage again. Continue to replace them until the wound

20   heals up.[82] *De methodo [medendi]* 5.[83]

(48) If you see that the medications are unable to dissolve the entire [quantity of] pus, but that the pus overpowers them and prevails over them, it is necessary to lance and incise the abscess at its highest and thinnest point. Let the pus flow out, and then put drying [medicines] on

25   it that do not have a biting effect. But if you find that part of the bodily part has putrefied, excising that which has putrefied is unavoidable. Sometimes you have to excise, from the skin of armpits and groins, something of the shape of a laurel leaf,[84] because of the slackness of the skin in these places. Take care that the direction[85] of the incision be in

30   the width of the groin, not in its length. After the incision, fill up the site with pulverized frankincense. *De methodo [medendi]* 13.[86]

(49) When humors become entangled in a part of the body that is between the homoiomerous parts[87] and have to be evacuated from that very part, one should [first] put medicines on that spot which repels

35   that which streams to it, and then one should evacuate them [the humors] through an incision and dissolving drugs—especially when you suspect that something [of those humors] is being retained in those spots that are between the homoiomerous parts. *De arte parva.*[88]

المثال متى عرض في المفصل من المفاصل الكبار خلع مع قرحة عالجنا القرحة حتّى يبرأ
وإن كان لا يمكن جبر الخلع بعد ذلك. لا تأتِ إن رمنا ردّ الخلع مع القرحة أصابته في أكثر
الأمر تشنّج فنداوي الأخطر. ثالثة الحيلة.

٤٧. هذا دواء يقطع الدم المنبعث ولو من الأوداج: تأخذ كندرأ أودقاق الكندر
٥ وصبر واخلطهما بياض البيض حتّى يصير الدواء في ثخانة العسل. وتلوث فيه وبر
أرنب وتضعه على العرق المخروق والجراحة بجملتها ولفّ عليه لفّا جيّدا. وتحفّظ من
الأوجاع لأنّه ليس في الدنيا أبلغ في تهيّج انبعاث الدم من الوجع. ثمّ حلّ الرباط بعد
ثلاثة أيّام فإن وجدت الدواء لا زما للجرح لزوما محكما فلا تقلعه وضع عليه من ذلك
الدواء كأنّك تندي به الوبر واربطه كالأولى وإن سقط الوبر فاعمل ثانيا واربطه
١٠ أيضا. ولا تزال تغيّر ذلك دائما حتّى ينبت. خامسة الحيلة.

٤٨. إذا رأيت الأدوية لا تقوى على تحليل القيح كلّه بل قهرها القيح وغلبها ينبغي
أن تبطّ الخراج وتشقّه في أعلى مكان فيه وأرقّه. ويسيل القيح واجعل ما يجفّف من
غير لذع. وإن وجدت شيئا من العضو قد عفن فلا بدّ من قطع ما عفن. وقد تحتاج
أن تقطع من جلد الإبطين والحالبين قدر ورقة آس لرخاوة جلدة هذه المواضع.
١٥ واجعل طول القطع ذاهبا في عرض الأربية لا في طولها. وبعد القطع تملأ الموضع من
دقاق الكندر. ثالثة عشر الحيلة.

٤٩. إذا ارتبكت الأخلاط في العضو بين الأعضاء المتشابهة الأجزاء ولزم
أن تستفرغ من العضو نفسه فينبغي أن تضع على ما فوق ذلك العضو أدوية تدفع ما يجري
إليه والاستفراغ يكون بالبطّ وبالأدوية المحلّلة ولا سيّما إن توهّمت أن في المواضع التي
٢٠ فيما بين الأعضاء المتشابهة الأجزاء شيئا محتبسا. في الصناعة الصغيرة.

---

٤ الكندر] G¹ || ٥ ثخانة] ثخن EL || ٦ والجراحة] والجرحة L || ١٢ وأرقّه] واحرقه
L || ١٣ ما عفن] G¹ || ١٧ ارتبكت] أكثرت L

(50) If you scarify bloody inflammations that occur without an external cause,[89] the one affected by it suffers from a grave affliction, especially
if you do so at the outset. But if the illness lasts for a long time, there is
no objection to scarification. Similarly, when the inflammation known as
5   *ḥumra*,[90] has reached the condition of lividness, greenness, or blackness,
it should be scarified. *Ad Glauconem [de methodo medendi]* 2.[91]

(51) [In the case of] the inflammation which is called *ḥumra*,[92] one
should, first of all, cool it. When its seething heat subsides,[93] scarification and the application of a poultice made from barley [*Hordeum vulgare*
10   and var.] meal and then heat is beneficial. *Ad Glauconem [de methodo
medendi]* 2.[94]

(52) If an inflamed tumor is difficult to suppurate and dissolve, and
the humors that got stuck in that part of the body contain a thick and
viscous superfluity, one should apply deep scarification. Also good for
15   these tumors is a cataplasm made of figs.[95] For this, one should boil the
figs until their moisture attains the consistency of bees' honey. Mix this
one time with barley meal and another time with bread from coarse
meal. *Ad Glauconem [de methodo medendi]* 2.[96]

(53) I found that superficial scarification is of little benefit and use in
20   the case of [inflamed tumors]. But an incision that is deep and extremely
long evacuates such a large quantity [of superfluities] that the patient
almost faints. Therefore, such an incision needs its own special treatment.[97]
But an incision intermediate between these two is free from these harmful effects. Therefore, I thought it a good thing to always employ this
25   [kind of incision] except [in the case of] the [inflamed tumor], which is
difficult to coct and dissolve. For then, one should resort to [making] a
deep incision. *Ad Glauconem [de methodo medendi]* 2.[98]

(54) Two [kinds of] superfluities necessarily develop in bodies: One
of them is thin and dissolves in a hidden way, and the other is thick; and
30   the latter is the filth that accumulates on the surface of a body. The
thin superfluity in an ulcer is called *ṣadīd*,[99] while the thick superfluity
in an ulcer is called *waḍar*.[100] An ulcer becomes moist or dirty because of
an excess of the thin or the thick secretion.[101] When an ulcer is moist, it

٥٠. الأورام الدموية التي تحدث من غير سبب من خارج متى شرطها كسبت صاحبها بلاء عظيما وخاصة إن فعلت ذلك أولا. أما إذا طالت العلة فلا بأس بالشرط. وكذلك الورم المعروف بالحمرة إذا آلت حاله إلى الكمودة أو الخضرة أو السواد فإنه يشرط. ثانية أغلوقن.

٥ ٥١. الورم الذي يسمى حمرة يستعمل التبريد في أول الأمر فإذا هدأت حرارته وبطل غليانه فينفعه الشرط والتضميد بضماد يتخذ بدقيق الشعير مسخن. ثانية أغلوقن.

٥٢. متى كان الورم عسر التقيح وعسر التحليل فالأخلاط التي لجت في ذلك العضو معها فضل غليظ ولزوجة فينبغي استعمال الشرط الغائر. ويصلح أيضا في هذه الأورام الضماد المتخذ بالتين وهو أن يطبخ التين حتى يصير لمائه قوام العسل المحل.

١٠ فتخلطه مرة بدقيق الشعير ومرة بالخبز الحشكار. ثانية أغلوقن.

٥٣. وجدت الشرط الذي ليس بغائر ضعيف النفع قليل الغناء في الأورام. والشرط الغائر الممعن في الطول يستفرغ كثيرا جدا حتى يكاد صاحبه يغشى عليه. ويحتاج ذلك الشرط بنفسه إلى علاج يخصه. والشرط الذي بين الشرطين سالما من الآفتين ولذلك رأيت استعماله دائما إلا في ما عسر نضجه وتحليله من الأورام.

١٥ فإنه يلتجأ إلى الشرط الغائر. ثانية أغلوقن.

٥٤. تتولد في الأبدان فضلتان ضرورة: إحداهما لطيفة تتحلل من البدن بالتحلل الخفي والأخرى غليظة هي الوسخ الذي يجتمع على البدن. وتلك اللطيفة في القرحة يقال لها صديدا وتلك الغليظة في القرحة وضرا. وتصير القرحة رطبة أو وضرة من كثرة إحدى هاتين الفضلتين. فتحتاج القرحة ضرورة من أجل رطوبتها

---

necessarily needs something that dries it up without biting, and when it is dirty, it necessarily needs something that cleanses it. In deep ulcers, the production of these two superfluities never stops, not even for one moment. *De methodo [medendi]* 3.[102]

(55) When an ulcer is deep, it always needs a drying and cleansing medication. A remedy that makes the flesh grow should be in the first grade of dryness, moderately drying and cleansing in the manner of frankincense, meal of barley, meal of beans, meal of bitter vetch, lily [*Lilium*][103] roots,[104] opopanax plant, tutty,[105] and wine,[106] [for these are] excellent remedies for all ulcers. *De methodo [medendi]* 3.[107]

(56) A remedy that closes a wound with flesh[108] should be more drying than a remedy that makes the flesh grow[109] and does not need the same cleansing and purifying action as a remedy that makes the flesh grow. Rather, a remedy that makes the flesh grow should be astringent. A remedy that seals a wound and promotes cicatrization should be more drying than a remedy that closes a wound with flesh, because the former has to dry and harden the surface of the flesh that has been formed in the wound. It has to dry it and to make it replace the skin. Such a remedy is unripe[110] gallnuts [of *Quercus* sp. and var.], pomegranate [*Punica granatum* and var.] peels, fruit of Egyptian thorn [*Acacia nilotica*],[111] rose or blossom of the wild pomegranate [*Punica granatum* l. and var.],[112] and the like. *De methodo [medendi]* 3.[113]

(57) The overgrowth of flesh in an ulcer needs a very drying remedy that also cleanses or eats away [the flesh], such as verdigris. *De methodo [medendi]* 3.[114]

(58) With many of those in [whose cases] you want to pour a medicine into their nose [as a treatment for a cold and lasting catarrh],[115] you should proceed as follows: Take nigella [*Nigella sativa* and var.], pulverize it until it becomes like dust, mix it with old olive oil, and pound it into a very fine substance. Then tell the patient to fill his mouth with water and to tilt his head back as far as possible, and pour this medicine into his nose and tell him to inhale so that he draws in the medicine more strongly. *De instrumento odoratus.*[116]

(59) The story goes about a man who suffered from a persistent ulcer on his thigh which was hard to heal. He went to an eminent physician,[117] who bled him from his arm and who, when he saw that his blood was black and thick, extracted a small amount of blood on the first day

إلى ما يجفّف من غير لذع ومن أجل وضرها إلى ما ينقّي. ولا ينقطع تولّد هاتين الفضلتين في القرحة الغائرة ولا وقت واحد. ثالثة الحيلة.

٥٥. القرحة الغائرة تحتاج دائمًا إلى دواء مجفّف ومنقّ. والدواء المنبت للحم ينبغي أن يكون في الدرجة الأولى من التجفيف معتدل التجفيف والتنقية بمنزلة الكندر ودقيق الشعير ودقيق الباقلّى ودقيق الكرسنة وأصول السوسن ونبات الجاوشير والتوتيا والشراب دواء جيّد لجميع القروح. ثالثة الحيلة.

٥٦. الدواء الملحم ينبغي أن يكون أشدّ تجفيفًا من المنبت للحم ولا يكون فيه جلاء وتنقية كما يحتاج إلى ذلك المنبت للحم. بل يكون الملحم مقبّضًا. والدواء الذي يختم ويدمل أزيد تجفيفًا من الدواء اللاحم لأنه يجفّف سطح اللحم الذي قد التحم ويصلّبه ويجفّفه ويجعله ينوب مناب الجلد. وذلك كالعفص الأخضر وقشور الرمّان والقرض والجلّنار ونحوها. ثالثة الحيلة.

٥٧. اللحم الزائد النابت في القرحة يحتاج إلى دواء يجفّف تجفيفًا أزيد ويجلو أو يأكل بمنزلة الزنيار. ثالثة الحيلة.

٥٨. كثير ممن تريد تسعطهم، تسعطهم على هذا المثال: يؤخذ شونيز فيدقّ حتى يصير كالغبار ويخلط بزيت عتيق ويسحق سحقًا ناعمًا. ثمّ تأمر العليل أن يملأ فه ماء وينكس رأسه إلى خلف بغاية ما يمكنه. ويسعط بهذا الدواء ويؤمر أن يتنفّس إلى داخل حتى يجذب الدواء بفضل قوة. في مقالته في آلة الشمّ.

٥٩. حكي عن رجل كان في فخذه قرحة مزمنة عسر بروءها. فأتى إلى طبيب فاضل ففصده في يده فرأى الدم اسود غليظًا فأخرج منه في اليوم الأوّل شيئًا قليلا

---

٣ للحم] om. EL ‖ ٥ وأصول] وأصل L ‖ ٦ ثالثة] عشر add. G ‖ ١٠ والقرض] والقرظ U ‖ ١٣ ثالثة الحيلة] في مقالته تلك EL ‖ ١٦ ويؤمر ... الدواء] G¹

[thereafter][118] and similarly on the third and fourth day. He then purged him three times with a medicine that evacuates the black chyme and fed him with nutriments producing good chymes. Then he turned to treating the ulcer itself, and it healed. *De atra bile.*[119]

5   (60) If you think it proper to make an incision but the patient is faint-hearted or it is distressing for his family, make him think that you are going to palpate or rub [the spot you want to incise] with oil, and then make the incision, so that you take him unawares. *De officina [medici]* 1.[120]

(61) There is no advantage in evacuating a humor that is going to 10 turn to pus, for it is a better and quicker way to ensure simultaneous change if one leaves it inside until the rest of what is within changes. *De officina [medici]* 2.[121]

(62) If a broken nasal bone is set, it will heal and grow together within ten days. [Broken] jaw, collarbone, and ribs[122] [heal] within twenty days. 15 A [broken] upper arm[123] [heals] within thirty days. A [broken] leg and forearm[124] [heal] within forty days. A [broken] thigh [heals] within fifty days. *In Hippocratem De alimento commentarius* 4.[125]

(63) [Broken] bones of young people heal sooner than those of children, because children need material for their growth to replace the 20 matter which has been dissolved. This was mentioned by Asklepios in the first treatise of his commentary on [Hippocrates'] book on [fractures] and their setting.[126]

(64) Do not attempt to set any broken bone if only four days have passed, lest you cause the patient severe harm. The third [treatise] of 25 Asklepios' commentary on [Hippocrates'] book on [fractures] and their setting.

(65) In the case of broken bones,[127] apply pads immersed in astringent dark wine, especially in the summer. For, if you use olive oil or cerate, putrefaction develops in [those] parts. *De methodo medendi* 6.[128]

وكذلك أخرج له في اليوم الثالث والرابع وأسهله بدواء يخرج الكيموس الأسود ثلاث مرّات وغذاه بأغذية جيّدة الكيموس. ثمة صار بعد ذلك إلى مداواة القرحة فبرأت. في مقالته في المرة السوداء.

٦٠. إذا حسن عندك أن تبطّ وكان المريض جبانا أو يشق ذلك على من حوله ٥ فأوهمه أنّك تغمز أوتدهن وتبطّه من حيث لا يشعر من قبل. في الأولى من الحانوت.

٦١. ليس ينتفع بخروج شيء من الخلط الذي يريد أن يصير مدّة لأنّ مكثه داخل إلى أن يتغيّر معه سائر ما هناك أجود وأسرع للتغيّر معا. في ثانية الحانوت.

٦٢. عظم الأنف ينجبر كسره ويصحّ ويلتئم في عشرة أيّام. فأمّا اللحي والترقوة والجنبين في عشرين يوما. وأمّا العضد في ثلاثين يوما وأمّا الساق والساعد في أربعين ١٠ يوما. وأمّا الفخذ في خمسين يوما. في رابعة من شرح الغذاء.

٦٣. العظام في الشابّ تنجبر قبل انجبارها في الفتيان لأنّ الفتيان يحتجون إلى مادّة ينموا بها وتخلّف ما يتحلّل منهم. ذكر ذلك أسقليبيوس في المقالة الأولى من شرحه لكتاب الجبر.

٦٤. كلّ عظم انكسر إذا مضى له أربعة أيام فلا زاد فلا ترم جبره لئلا تجلب على المريض مضرّة عظيمة. في الثالثة من شرح أسقليبيوس لكتاب الجبر. ١٥

٦٥. عند كسر العظام اجعل الرفائد مغموسة في شراب قابض أسود وخاصّة في الصيف. فإنّك إذا استعملت في الصيف الزيت أو القير وطلي حدث في الأعضاء عفونة. سادسة الحيلة.

---

١ اليوم] الثاني و– add.B || ٦ ليس ... الحانوت [om.B : G¹ || ٨ كسره] بثره L | اللحي و–] om.EL || ١٠ وأمّا الفخذ في خمسين يوما [om.EL : U¹ || ١١ الشابّ] الشباب ELBOU || ١٢ مادّة] مذة G | أسقليبيوس] أسقليوس EL || ١٥ في الثالثة من شرح أسقليبيوس لكتاب الجبر] من ذلك الكتاب EL || ١٨ سادسة الحيلة] G¹ : ثالثة الحيلة G

(66) In the case of fractures and ulcers, the patient should feel more pressure of the bandage on the affected spot [itself] and less on the extremities. But a bandage with which one intends to increase the flesh of an emaciated limb should be as slack as possible on the emaciated limb itself and exert its greatest pressure on the sound parts nearby, so that blood is admitted to the emaciated limb. *De officina [medici]* 3.[129]

(67) When you set the arm or leg, place it in the position customary for that patient. For there are some people whose legs are stretched during the entire day, while there are others whose legs are flexed. *De officina [medici]* 3.[130]

(68) Fractures of the leg require a cast,[131] so that the limb is not troubled during moving. You should carefully investigate the injuries which require a cast, for if the harm caused by the cast is greater than its benefit, do not apply it. *De officina [medici]* 3.[132]

(69) [In cases of fracture], first put a bandage under the pads. Begin from the spot of the injury and end higher up to prevent moistures from streaming [to that part] so that it does not become inflamed. Then apply the pads; and then put a bandage on top of the pads, so that they do not become disordered, beginning with the spot of the injury and ending downward in order to force the putrid blood from the injured limb to its extremity. After this second bandage, apply the trusses which secure and support all that is behind [them]. Thus, there are four things that surround the limb: the bandage that has contact with the limb, the pads, the bandage on these, and the trusses. *De officina [medici]* 3.[133]

٦٦. ينبغي أن يكون المريض يجد مسّ ضغط الرباط في موضع العلّة أكثر وفي الطرفين أقلّ، هذا في حال الكسر والقرحة. وأمّا الرباط الذي يرام به تسمين العضو المهزول فأرخى ما يكون على العضو المهزول وأشدّ ما يكون على ما يليه من الأعضاء السليمة لينبعث الدم إلى العضو المهزول. في ثالثة الحانوت.

٦٧. إذا جبرت يدا أو رجلا فاجعل شكل وضعها الشكل الذي جرت العادة به دائما لذلك الشخص. فمن الناس من رجله مبسوطة نهاره أجمع ومنهم من هي منه مقبوضة. في ثالثة الحانوت.

٦٨. كسور الرجل تحتاج إلى قالب لئلا يضطرب العضو عند الحركة. وينبغي أن تنعم النظر في المرض الموجب القالب، فإن كانت المضارّ التي تحدث من القالب أكثر من منافعه فلا تستعمل. في ثالثة الحانوت.

٦٩. ينبغي أن تربط أولا تحت الرفائد وتبدأ من موضع العلّة وتنتهي إلى الموضع الأعلى لتمنع انصباب الرطوبات فيمنع التورّم. ثمّ تجعل الرفائد، ثمّ تربط من فوق الرفائد كلا تتشوّش وتبتدئ من موضع العلّة وتنتهي إلى أسفل ليعصر الدم العفن من العضو العليل إلى الطرف. وبعد هذا الرباط الثاني تجعل الجبائر وهي تشكّل ما هو وراءها وتدعمه. فيكون جميع ما يحوط بالعضو أربعة أشياء: الرباط الذي يلقى العضو والرفائد والرباط الذي عليها والجبائر. في ثالثة الحانوت.

---

٣ فأرخي] فاحرى (!)G ‖ ٨ أن تنعم النظر في المرض الموجب القالب] om. L ‖ ١٢ فيمنع] فيشع ELBU ‖ ١٤ وهي تشكّل ما هو وراءها وتدعمه] وهي ألتي تسند تلك كلّها وتدعمها

Ibn Ridwān, *Compendium of Galen's commentary on Hippocrates' KAT' IHTREION*, ed. Lyons, p. 114, l. 10–11.

(70) The pads should be placed on the thinnest part of the limb so as to make it level with the thick part, so that when it is secured by a bandage, the pressure exerted may be even. For if it is not even, the bandage will work loose. The width of the bandage should be three[134] thumbs. *De officina [medici]* 3.[135]

This is the end of the fifteenth treatise,
by the grace of God, praise be to Him.

◆

٧٠. ينبغي أن تجعل الرفائد في الموضع الأرق من العضو حتى يعتدل مع الغليظ وتشده بالرباط فيقع الشد مستويا فإنه إن اختلف استرخى. ويكون عرض العصابة ثلاثة أصابع. في ثالثة الحانوت.

تمت المقالة الخامسة عشر ولله الحمد والمنة.

---

٤ تمت المقالة الخامسة عشر ولله الحمد والمنة] كملت المقالة الخامسة عشر والحمد لله كثيرا وعدد فصولها تسعة وشتين E: تمت المقالة الخامسة عشر وعدد فصولها تسعة وشتين فصلا L: تمت B: تمت المقالة الخامسة عشر الحمد لله وعدد فصولها تسعة وشتين O: تمت المقالة السابعة وعدد فصولها تسعة وشتين U

Supplement

Critical comparison of the Arabic text with the
Hebrew translations and the translation into English

10.3: فتوخّ ما يبقي القوة ويرفدها (set your mind on that which maintains and supports the strength): Reading فتوخّ as فتوقّ, **N** translates: יזהר מה שנשאר מן הכח ותסעדהו, and **r**: "be careful about the remaining (body) strength and support it." **Z** translates فتوخّ as עשה.

10.22: وليس فيها لذاذة أصلا (nothing at all is pleasant about it): **N** translates لذاذة as הנחה, probably in the sense of הנחת רוח (pleasure). However, **r**, understanding it more literally, translates: "It does not let up at all." **Z** provides a better translation: ערבות.

10.29: كأنّ العظام ترضّ بالثلج (as if his bones were being crushed by snow): **N**, reading العظام as العطس (sneezing) and ترضّ as يبرد (to cool), translates: יהיה העטוש מקרר כשלג. Accordingly, **r** translates: "that sneezing is as cold as snow." **Z** translates correctly: כאלו העצמות מתרוצצות בשלג.

10.37: النافض الذي لا يسكن (the rigor which does not abate): Reading لا يسكن as لا يسخن, **N** translates: הרתת אשר לא יחמם, which is translated by **r** as "Chills which do not warm." **Z** reads the text just like **N** and translates: הפלצות אשר לא יחום.

10.37: والضرب الآخر هو الذي لا يسكن (There are two kinds of rigor that do not abate): Reading لا يسكن as لا يسخن, **N** translates: והמין האחר אותו שלא יתחמם, which is translated by **r** as "The other type does not warm."

Z, reading the text just like **N**, translates: והפנים האחרות אשר לא יחום. Following the reading by MS **L**: والضرب الآخر هو الذي يسخن, Deller translates: "Die zweite Art wird erhitzt."

10.40: الحميّات المحرقة لا يكاد تتولّد من (Ardent fevers hardly ever originate from): Reading يكاد as لا يظنّ, **N** translates: לא יחשב שתולד מן, and **r**, following **N**: "One should not assume that burning fever develops." **Z** translates: הקדחות השורפות אינם נולדות מן (ardent fevers do not develop from).

10.40: احتقان (congestion): Reading احتقان as احتراق, **N** translates: שרפה, and **r**, following **N**: "burning." **Z** translates correctly: העצר.

10.40: الهواء (the air): Reading this term as الجهد, **N** translates: העמל, and **r**: "work." **Z** translates correctly: אויר.

10.45: اختلاف نيء (diarrhea of raw material): Reading نيء as قيء, Deller translates: "Erbrechen."

10.54: كل مكان من الأمراض يهيج وينوب على الأدوار (Any illness that flares up and attacks in cycles): The term يهيج has been correctly translated by **N** as שיעור. However, **m** has misread it as שיעורה, and this results in **r**'s translation: "Any illness which has a limit and whose episodes occur in cycles."

10.57: مستوقد الحمّى (the hearth of the fever): Not reading مستوقد but مستودع, **N** translates: מנוח and **r**, following **N**: "focus" (cf. **r**, n. 107: lit., "resting place"). **Z** translates correctly: יוקדת.

10.68: ولا تغذوهم ولو في انحطاط النوبة (Do not feed them—not even when the [fever] attack abates): **N** translates the particle ولو incorrectly as אלא (but). This mistake probably goes back to a scribal error, as the correct translation, ולא, features in MS Munich 287, fol. 63a. The faulty reading is the basis for **r**: "Feed him only when the fever decreases." **Z** translates correctly: ולא.

11.15: قد يكون بحران يوثق بصحّته في علل الرأس (In the case of diseases of the head, a certainly safe crisis): Reading بصحّته as: صاحبه, **N** and **Z** translate: בעליו (those suffering from it), and **r**: "Sometimes in head illness the crisis alleviates the patient."

11.24: وقد يسمّى أيضا حادّا ما عرض من النكس (The illness occurring from a relapse is also called acute): Both **N** and **Z** misinterpret the Arabic النكس, **N** translating it as גשם (substance, body) and **Z** as נפש (= نفس). Following **N**, **r** translates: "Sometimes one uses the name "acute" to denote (the acuteness) of the substance (causing the illness)." **Bo** translates the term correctly as "recidivatio" (relapse).

12.18: وتفقد أيضا حمية خروج الدم إذا انقطعت (You should also pay attention to a reduction in the intensity of the flow of the blood): Reading حمية (gravity, vehemence) as حمية (abstention), **N** translates: ובדוק גם כן שמירת יציאת הדם כשתפסק and **r**: "Also examine the sediment of the extruded blood after (the phlebotomy) has terminated. **Z** does not translate the term حمية. **Bo** translates the term correctly as "furiositas."

12.22: الصرع (epilepsy): Reading الصداع (headache) instead of الصرع (epilepsy), **N** translates it as כאב הראש, and **r** as "cephalalgia." **Z** translates it correctly as הוויציאו הוא אלצרע (cf. aphorisms 7.29 and 9.23).

12.26: فصد المحموم (bleeding someone suffering from a fever): Possibly reading المحموم as المسموم, **N** translates: בעל הארס (someone who has been poisoned), and **r**: "a person who requires a phlebotomy." **Z** translates correctly: המוקדח.

12.45: متى داويت صلابة الطحال (When you treat hardness of the spleen): Reading داويت as رأيت, **N** translates: כשראית קשי הטחול, and **r**: "If you observe hardness of the spleen." **Z** translates correctly: כשתרפא קושי הטחול.

13.6: خمل المعدة (the lining of the stomach): **N** translates correctly: קמטי האצטומכה. However, **Z** translates incorrectly: יחריב האצט' (destroys the stomach).

13.9: المرة الصفراء يسهل استفراغها بأهون سعي (Yellow bile can be evacuated with minimal effort): Reading سعي (effort) as سعة (width), **N** translates: המרה האדומה יקל הרקתה בהרחבה נקלה, and **r**: "Red bile is easy to eliminate since it facilitates widening (of excretory passageways)." **Z** translates بأهون سعي as בנקלה (easily).

13.36: وبما من شأنه أن يغري ويلصق ([one should apply an enema] with that whose property it is . . . to have an agglutinant and cohesive effect): Reading يغري as يجري, **N** translates: ובמה שדרכו להזיל ולהמעיד. This is translated by **r** as: "and that (also) liquifies the intestinal contents." **Z** translates correctly: ובמה שדרכו שידבק ויחבר.

13.51: حجاب شحم الحنظل (The rind [enclosing] the pulp of colocynth): **N** translates correctly: מסך בשר הקולוקנטידא. However, **m**, understanding מסך as a transcription of the Arabic مسك (musk), emendates it as מור ("myrrh," but also interpreted as "musk"). And **r**, misunderstanding both **N** and **m**, translates: "myrtle fruit meat." **Z** translates حجاب as: תיקון (cf. **Bo:** "preparatio").

15.15: جراحة (wound): **N** translates this term correctly as חבורה, but **Z**, reading خراجة, translates: יציאה.

15.15: معرق معرّى من اللحم (free from flesh): Not interpreting معرق as a synonym for من معرّى in the sense of "free from," but as derived from عرق (vessel), **N** translates: עורק, and **r**: "vessel." **Z** understands the term correctly as a synonym and does not translate it.

15.19: اللحم الرخو المخلوق لحشو الفرج (the soft flesh created to fill up empty space): The terms لحشو الفرج are correctly translated by **N** as למלאת הפנאי, but misinterpreted by **Z** as להיותו מוצק לזולתו.

15.29: بمقدار يبرأ فيه الناصور (that the fistula in it [i.e., the eye] is cured): Reading يبرأ (is cured) as يبدأ (begins), **N** translates it as שיתחיל בה הנאצור, which is translated by **r** as "because a fistula might develop." This section is missing in **Bo** and **Z**.

15.36: سير (thong): Not reading سير but سيد, **N** translates: סיד (quicklime), and **r**: "lime water." **Z** translates correctly: רצועה.

15.39: ما . . . . يلصق (something that . . . agglutinates): Possibly reading يلصق as ينصق, **Z** translates: דבר שימעט (something that diminishes), while **N** translates it correctly as מה שידביק.

15.68: القالب (cast): **N** translates the term correctly as הדפוס, but **Z**, reading القلب instead of القالب, translates it as הלב (the heart).

Notes to the English Translation

The Tenth Treatise

1. "with astringent things": Not in Galen, *De methodo medendi* 11.15 (ed. Kühn, 10:788).
2. Galen, *De methodo medendi* 11.15 (ed. Kühn, 10:788).
3. Cf. Galen, *De methodo medendi* 9.5 (ed. Kühn, 10:622): ἐρυσίπελας δὲ τὸ γοῦν ἀκριβὲς οὐκ ἂν ἄλλως ἰάσαιο.
4. Galen, *De methodo medendi* 9.5 (ed. Kühn, 10:622).
5. "the most important": Lit., the beginning and the end.
6. "it is very good": Lit., that [is it].
7. Galen, *De methodo medendi* 10.1 (ed. Kühn, 10:662–65).
8. "of fevers": Cf. Galen, *De methodo medendi* 10.10 (ed. Kühn, 10:715): "of those suffering from fever" (ιῶν πυρcττόντων),
9. Galen, *De methodo medendi* 10.10 (ed. Kühn, 10:715–16).
10. "inflammation": Cf. Galen, *De methodo medendi* 10.10 (ed. Kühn, 10:716): φλεγμονή.
11. Galen, *De methodo medendi* 10.10 (ed. Kühn, 10:716).
12. "a fever patient": Cf. Galen, *In Hippocratis De acutorum morborum victu et Galeni commentarius* 1.32 (ed. Helmreich [CMG 5.9.1], 151 line 4): κάμνοντος.
13. Galen, *In Hippocratis De acutorum morborum victu et Galeni commentarius* 1.32 (ed. Helmreich [CMG 5.9.1], 151 lines 4–6).
14. Galen, *De differentiis febrium* 2.16 (ed. Kühn, 7:395–96).
15. "contraction of the [pulsatile] vessels [of the wrist]": Cf. Galen, *De differentiis febrium* 1.9 (ed. Kühn, 7:308): τῆς σφυγμῶν συστολῆς.
16. Galen, *De differentiis febrium* 1.9 (ed. Kühn, 7:308).
17. Cf. Galen, *Ad Glauconem de methodo medendi* 1.15 (ed. Kühn, 11:43): ἀλλ' οὐδὲ χρῄζει τινὸς ἄλλης κενώσεως.
18. "degree": Lit., amount.
19. Galen, *Ad Glauconem de methodo medendi* 1.15 (ed. Kühn, 11:43). The fourteenth-century French surgeon Guy de Chauliac refers to the Latin translation of this remedy for strengthening vision in his *Inventarium sive chirurgia magna*. Cf. Guigonis de Caulhiaco (Guy de Chauliac), *Inventarium sive chirurgia magna*, 1:393 lines 34–37, 2:330.

20. Galen, *Ad Glauconem de methodo medendi* 1.15 (ed. Kühn, 11:42–43).
21. "swollen glands": Cf. Galen, *De differentiis febrium* 1.7 (ed. Kühn, 7:297): βουβῶνες; Ullmann, *Wörterbuch zu den griechisch-arabischen*, 167–68.
22. Galen, *De differentiis febrium* 1.7 (ed. Kühn, 7:296–97); Cf. Maimonides, *Medical Aphorisms* 25.73 (ed. and trans. Bos, forthcoming).
23. "in the middle part of the body": Cf. Galen, *In Hippocratis Aphorismos commentarius* 7.26 (ed. Kühn, 18A:125): ἐν τοῖς μέσοις του σώματος.
24. "because of fainting or syncope": Cf. Galen, *In Hippocratis Aphorismos commentarius* 7.26 (ed. Kühn, 18A:125): διὰ λειποψυχίαν; Ullmann, *Wörterbuch zu den griechisch-arabischen*, 385, s.v. λειποψυχέω.
25. "drowning and choking effect": Cf. Galen, *In Hippocratis Aphorismos commentarius* 7.26 (ed. Kühn, 18A:125): πνίγεσθαι; Ullmann, *Wörterbuch zu den griechisch-arabischen*, 541, s.v. πνίγω.
26. Galen, *In Hippocratis Aphorismos commentarius* 7.26 (ed. Kühn, 18A:124–25).
27. Galen, *In Hippocratis Prognostica commentarius* 2.4 (ed. Kühn, 18B:119–21).
28. Galen, *In Hippocratis Epidemiarum* 3.2 (ed. Wenkebach [CMG 5.10.2.1], 74 lines 24–26; Deller translation, 529, no. 46).
29. This work of doubtful authenticity does not feature in the lists of works composed by Galen or ascribed to him. Cf. translator's introduction to Maimonides, *Medical Aphorisms* (ed. and trans. Bos, 1:xxi); Maimonides, *Medical Aphorisms* 3.76, 6.24 (ed. and trans. Bos, 1:52; 2:6).
30. "This putrefaction is to the fever as a blazing fire": Added by Maimonides.
31. Galen, *De methodo medendi* 11.4 (ed. Kühn, 10:744).
32. Galen, *De methodo medendi* 11.9 (ed. Kühn, 10:757–58).
33. "differentiation": Lit., comparison.
34. Galen, *De methodo medendi* 11.9 (ed. Kühn, 10:758).
35. Galen, *De methodo medendi* 12.3 (ed. Kühn, 10:821–22).
36. Galen, *De differentiis febrium* 2.1–2 (ed. Kühn, 7:336); cf. Maimonides' *Epitome*, MS Paris 1203, fols. 9a–b; Maimonides, *Medical Aphorisms* 25.23 (ed. and trans. Bos, forthcoming); Langermann, *Synochous Fever*, 187.
37. Namely, yellow bile, phlegm, black bile; see previous aphorism.
38. Galen, *De differentiis febrium* 2.1, 7 (ed. Kühn, 7:336, 354–55); cf. Maimonides, *Medical Aphorisms* 25.23 (ed. and trans. Bos, forthcoming).
39. I.e., to go through its different phases. Cf. Galen, *De diebus decretoriis* 2.12 (ed. Kühn, 9:888): μη παυόμενον εἰς ἀπυρεξίαν.
40. Galen, *De diebus decretoriis* 2.12 (ed. Kühn, 9:888–89).
41. "in a very obscure way": Cf. Galen, *De differentiis febrium* 1.9 (ed. Kühn, 7:308): ἀμυδρὰ.
42. Galen, *De differentiis febrium* 1.9 (ed. Kühn, 7:306–8).
43. I.e., when the blood putrefies.
44. Galen, *De differentiis febrium* 2.11 (ed. Kühn, 7:376–77).
45. I.e., quotidian fever caused by phlegm. Cf. Galen, *De circuitibus febrium* 4 (ed. Kühn, 7:494): ἀμφημερινός.
46. Galen, *De circuitibus febrium* 4 (ed. Kühn, 7:494).
47. Galen, *Ad Glauconem de methodo medendi* 1.2 (ed. Kühn, 11:9–10).
48. Galen, *De differentiis febrium* 2.18 (ed. Kühn, 7:404).

49. Galen, *De crisibus* 1.3 (ed. Kühn, 9:553–54; ed. Alexanderson, 70–71).

50. Galen, *De crisibus* 2.3 (ed. Kühn, 9:652–55; ed. Alexanderson, 133–35).

51. *De crisibus* 2.3 (ed. Kühn, 9:652–53; ed. Alexanderson, 133–34).

52. *De crisibus* 2.5 (ed. Kühn, 9:660–61; ed. Alexanderson, 138–39).

53. *De crisibus* 2.6, 12 (ed. Kühn, 9:664, 693; ed. Alexanderson, 141, 160).

54. "to rarefy contracted spots of the skin": Cf. Galen, *De methodo medendi* 11.4 (ed. Kühn, 10:747): ἀραιοῦν τὰ πεπυκνώμενα.

55. Galen, *De methodo medendi* 11.4 (ed. Kühn, 10:747).

56. Galen, *Ad Glauconem de methodo medendi* 1.10 (ed. Kühn, 11:32–33).

57. "I do not know that I [ever] saw": Cf. Galen, *Ad Glauconem de medendi methodo* 1.10 (ed. Kühn, 11:32–33): οὐκ οἴδαμεν. Although in this context the Greek means "I did not see," the Arabic translator preserved both possible meanings of the Greek, namely, to see and to know.

58. "the fever called 'the mixed one'": Cf. Galen, *Ad Glauconem de medendi methodo* 1.5 (ed. Kühn, 11:18): τοῖς καλουμένοις πλάνησι τε καὶ πλανήταις ("fevers called 'planetes,'" i.e., those that come in irregular fits).

59. Galen, *Ad Glauconem de methodo medendi* 1.5 (ed. Kühn, 11:18).

60. Galen, *Ad Glauconem de methodo medendi* 1.9 (ed. Kühn, 11:26).

61. Galen, *De inequali intemperie* 8 (ed. Kühn, 7:749–50). For a comparison between the Galenic text in the translation by Ḥunayn, as extant in MS Ayasofya 3593, fol. 52a, see introduction.

62. "malignant": Cf. Galen, *In Hippocratis Epidemiarum* 6.1 (ed. Wenkebach and Pfaff [CMG 5.10.2.2], 31 line 9): κακοηθέστερον.

63. Galen, *In Hippocratis Epidemiarum* 6.1 (ed. Wenkebach and Pfaff [CMG 5.10.2.2], 30 line 25–31 line 14; translation Deller, 532, no. 62).

64. Galen, *De differentiis febrium* 2.3, 10 (ed. Kühn, 7:339, 372).

65. Galen, *De crisibus* 2.2 (ed. Kühn, 9:646; ed. Alexanderson, 129 lines 22–25).

66. "from the domination of the heat": Cf. Galen, *In Hippocratis Epidemiarum* 1.2 (ed. Wenkebach and Pfaff [CMG 5.10.1], 59 line 11): τῆς θερμασίας ἀπεκταθείσης (from the heat drawn off).

67. "through the condition of the air": Cf. Galen, *In Hippocratis Epidemiarum* 1.2 (ed. Wenkebach and Pfaff [CMG 5.10.1], 59 line 13): ἐν ἡλίῳ διατρίψασιν ([as happens in the case of] those who spend too much time in the sun).

68. *In Hippocratis Epidemiarum* 1.2 (ed. Wenkebach and Pfaff [CMG 5.10.1], 59 lines 9–15; Deller translation, 521, no. 5).

69. "similar to a smoldering fire": Cf. Galen, *Ad Glauconem de methodo medendi* 1.16 (ed. Kühn, 11:65): οἶον σμυχόμενοι.

70. Galen, *Ad Glauconem de methodo medendi* 1.16 (ed. Kühn, 11:65).

71. Galen, *De locis affectis* 5.7 (ed. Kühn 8:348; trans. Siegel, 156).

72. Galen, *In Hippocratis Epidemiarum* 1.1 (ed. Wenkebach and Pfaff [CMG 5.10.1], 41 lines 12–15; Deller translation, 521, no. 3).

73. Galen, *In Hippocratis Epidemiarum* 2.2 (ed. Wenkebach and Pfaff [CMG 5.10.1], 252 lines 25–29; Deller translation, 521, no. 3).

74. Galen, *In Hippocratis Epidemiarum* 3.2 (ed. Wenkebach [CMG 5.10.2.1], 98 lines 13–20; Deller translation, 530, no. 47).

75. "a blazing heat so intense that it can be felt through touching": Cf. Galen, *In Hippocratis Epidemiarum* 3.3 (ed. Wenkebach [CMG 5.10.2.1], 132 line 19): θερμασίας διακαιούσης αἰσθανομένων τῶν καμνόντων.

76. Galen, *In Hippocratis Epidemiarum* 3.3 (ed. Wenkebach [CMG 5.10.2.1], 132 lines 17–19).

77. This text does not feature in Galen, *De methodo medendi* 12, but in *De methodo medendi* 11 (ed. Kühn, 10:759).

78. "ascends and rises": See Galen, *In Hippocratis Epidemiarum* 1.1 (ed. Wenkebach and Pfaff [CMG 5.10.1], 29 line 34): ἀναφερομένου; cf. **GB**: "boils and rises."

79. Galen, *In Hippocratis Epidemiarum* 1.1 (ed. Wenkebach and Pfaff [CMG 5.10.1], 29 lines 26–34).

80. Galen, *In Hippocratis de acutorum morborum victu liber et Galeni commentarius* 3 (ed. Helmreich [CMG 5.9.1], 267 line 28–268 line 3).

81. "unless it occurs in the beginning of the [fever] attacks": Added by Maimonides.

82. Galen, *In Hippocratis Epidemiarum* 2.3 (ed. Wenkebach and Pfaff [CMG 5.10.1], 258 lines 35–39).

83. Galen, *De methodo medendi* 11.9 (ed. Kühn, 10:760).

84. This Pseudo-Galenic treatise is perhaps identical with *Maqālah fī l-ḥuqan wa-l-qūlanj* (*De clysteribus et colica*) cited by Ibn Abī Uṣaybiᶜa, ᶜUyūn al-anbāʾ, 1.102; cf. Meyerhof, "Schriften Galens," 543, no. 62; Sezgin, *Medizin-Pharmazie*, 3:128, no. 100; Maimonides, *Medical Aphorisms* 7.65 (ed. and trans. Bos, 2:39).

85. Galen, *De differentiis febrium* 2.6 (ed. Kühn, 7:304; 349–50).

86. Galen, *De differentiis febrium* 2.18 (ed. Kühn, 7:404).

87. Galen, *De differentiis febrium* 2.18 (ed. Kühn, 7:404–5). This section is found only in MSS **G** and **U**.

88. Galen, *De crisibus* 1.3 (ed. Kühn, 9:552–53; ed. Alexanderson, 70 lines 18–20).

89. Galen, *De Theriaca ad Pisonem* (ed. Kühn, 14:15, 277); Richter-Bernburg, *De Theriaca ad Pisonem* (Arabic trans.), 125a:13–18. "Ad Pisonem": the Arabic title *ilā Qayṣar* is a corruption of *ilā Fīṣun*; cf. Steinschneider, *Griechischen Ärzte*, 292 (344), no. 55; Ullmann, *Medizin im Islam*, 49, no. 51. Nathan's Hebrew translation of this text is quoted in the name of Maimonides in a treatise on fever composed by Salmias (Salamias) of Lunel (MS Oxford, Bodleian, Marsh 347, Uri 422, Neubauer 2133, fols. 45a–b); cf. Gross, *Gallia Judaica*, 288–89, no. 25.

90. Galen, *De marcore liber* 7 (ed. Kühn, 7:692–93).

91. Galen, *De febribus* 1.11–13 (ed. Kühn, 7:321–22, 328).

92. This quotation is perhaps an adaptation of Galen, *In Hippocratis Epidemiarum* 3.3 (ed. Wenkebach [CMG 5.10.2.1], 163 lines 17–19). It is not quoted by Deller.

93. "I do not know that I [ever] saw": Cf. Galen, *De methodo medendi* 10.8 (ed. Kühn, 10:699): οὐκ εἶδον; cf. aphorism 10.34 above.

94. Galen, *De methodo medendi* 10.8 (ed. Kühn, 10:699).

95. "the main organs": Cf. Galen, *De methodo medendi* 10.11 (ed. Kühn, 10:729): τὰ στερεὰ (the solid parts).

96. Galen, *De methodo medendi* 10.11 (ed. Kühn, 10:729–30).
97. "to the type of fevers that cause the body to waste": Cf. Galen, *De methodo medendi* 10.11 (ed. Kühn, 10:731): ἐκ τοῦ τῶν συντηκόντων γένους.
98. Galen, *De methodo medendi* 10.11 (ed. Kühn, 10:731–32).
99. Galen, *De methodo medendi* 9.5 (ed. Kühn, 10:622–24); cf. Maimonides' *Epitome*, MS Paris 1203, fols. 81a–82a; Langermann, Synochous Fever, 184–85.
100. "For if he cools [him] down, he destroys [him]": Langermann, *Synochous Fever*, 184, translates: "he wrongly thought that he cooled the patient down."
101. Galen, *De methodo medendi* 9.5 (ed. Kühn, 10:619); cf. Maimonides' *Epitome*, MS Paris 1203, fols. 81a–b; Langermann, *Synochous Fever*, 184–85.
102. Galen, *De methodo medendi* 9.4 (ed. Kühn, 10:616); the Maimonidean text is a fairly accurate quotation and not a radical reformulation, as Langermann, *Synochous Fever*, 185, suggests.
103. Galen, *De methodo medendi* 9.2 (ed. Kühn, 10:604–5); cf. Maimonides' *Epitome*, MS Paris 1203, fol. 79b; Langermann, *Synochous Fever*, 185.
104. Galen, *De methodo medendi* 8.4 (ed. Kühn, 10:564–67).
105. "later": Lit., present.
106. Galen, *De methodo medendi* 8.5 (ed. Kühn, 10:571–72).
107. Galen, *De methodo medendi* 10.5 (ed. Kühn, 10:689).
108. Galen, *De methodo medendi* 11.5 (ed. Kühn, 10:749).
109. Galen, *De methodo medendi* 11.8 (ed. Kühn, 10:754).
110. Galen, *De methodo medendi* 11.21 (ed. Kühn, 10:808).

The Eleventh Treatise

1. "It is only with great toil that one can come to know the actual period of a disease at a certain moment through an exact conjecture": Cf. Galen, *De crisibus* 1.2 (ed. Kühn, 9:552; ed. Alexanderson, 70 lines 10–11): μόλις γὰρ ἂν οὕτως τις ἀκριβῆ στοχασμὸν ποιήσαι το τοῦ καθεστῶτος καιροῦ.
2. Galen, *De crisibus* 1.2 (ed. Kühn, 9:551–52; ed. Alexanderson, 69 lines 9–10, 70 lines 10–11).
3. "We . . . epilepsy": Cf. Maimonides, *Medical Aphorisms* 25.45 (ed. and trans. Bos, forthcoming).
4. Cf. Galen, *De totius morbi temporibus* 4 (ed. Kühn, 7:451): "nor should one describe apoplexy as the disease that particularly attacks very suddenly in full vigor. This is not exactly so, for although it passes through the stages of beginning and increase in a short time, it is not without a beginning, nor does it come on in an utterly perfect way, just as an attack of epilepsy does not. For no one is so suddenly seized by its symptoms as someone whose head is cut off, although even here the cutting takes a first, second, third, or fourth moment of time, no matter how the surgeon cuts."
5. "the four periods": I.e., beginning, increase, climax, and decline.
6. Galen, *De totius morbi temporibus* 4 (ed. Kühn, 7:451).
7. Galen, *De crisibus* 1.20 (ed. Kühn, 9:636–37; ed. Alexanderson, 124).

8. This text does not feature in Galen, *De morborum temporibus*, but in Galen, *De totius morbi temporibus* 4 (ed. Kühn, 7:453–54).

9. Just as in the previous case, this text does not show up in Galen, *De morborum temporibus*, but in Galen, *De totius morbi temporibus* 4 (ed. Kühn, 7:452–53).

10. Galen, *De crisibus* 1.3 (ed. Kühn, 9:557; ed. Alexanderson, 73).

11. "hidden, weak signs": Cf. Galen, *De crisibus* 1.17 (ed. Kühn, 9:625; ed. Alexanderson, 116 line 14): τὰ ἀμυδρὰ [σημεῖα].

12. Galen, *De crisibus* 1.17 (ed. Kühn, 9:624–25; ed. Alexanderson, 115 lines 21–23, 116 lines 13–14).

13. "A sign": Lit., signs.

14. "bright": Lit., saturated. Cf. Galen, *De crisibus* 1.17 (ed. Kühn, 9:625; ed. Alexanderson, 116 line 18): τὸ πυρρόν.

15. Galen, *De crisibus* 1.17 (ed. Kühn, 9:625; ed. Alexanderson, 116 lines 16–20).

16. "or urine that is moderately thick [and] has a healthy color but no sediment is a clear sign indicating the beginning of the increase [of the disease]": Lit., "or urine that is moderately thick with a healthy color is a clear sign indicating the beginning of the increase [of the disease] and the lack of sediment." The contradictory text has been corrected according to Galen, *De crisibus* 1.17 (ed. Kühn, 9:626): καὶ χωρὶς ὑποστάσεως δὲ τὸ εὔχρουν οὖρον ἅμα τῷ συμμέτρῳ πάχει πεπαῦσθαι δηλοῖ τὴν ἀρχήν.

17. Galen, *De crisibus* 1.17 (ed. Kühn, 9:625–26; ed. Alexanderson, 116 lines 20–24).

18. "inflamed tumors that are quick to move": Cf. Galen, *De crisibus* 2.11 (ed. Kühn, 9:690; ed. Alexanderson, 157 line 15): εὐκίνητοι καὶ θερμαὶ διαθέσεις.

19. Galen, *De crisibus* 2.11 (ed. Kühn, 9:690; ed. Alexanderson, 157 lines 12–15).

20. Galen, *De crisibus* 3.4 (ed. Kühn, 9:717; ed. Alexanderson, 177).

21. Galen, *De crisibus* 3.5 (ed. Kühn, 9:724–25; ed. Alexanderson, 181–82).

22. "that the crisis is announced beforehand on a day bordering on the crisis": Cf. Galen, *De crisibus* 3.3 (ed. Kühn, 9:706; ed. Alexanderson, 169 lines 21–22): τὸ προδεδηλῶσθαι διά τινος τῶν ἐπιδήλων, ᾗ συνῆπται τῆς κρινούσης ἡμέρας ἡ δύναμις ("The second is if the crisis has been previously announced by means of one of the clear [signs] with which is linked the force of the day that is the crisis"—i.e., if the crisis arrives, then it is supposed to arrive, and you have already foretold it.)

23. "the nature and way": Cf. Galen, *De crisibus* 3.3 (ed. Kühn, 9:707; ed. Alexanderson, 170 line 2): ἰδέαν.

24. Galen, *De crisibus* 3.3 (ed. Kühn, 9:706–7; ed. Alexanderson, 169–70).

25. "congenial to": I.e., good for; cf. Galen, *De crisibus* 3.3 (ed. Kühn, 9:708; ed. Alexanderson, 171 line 5): οἰκεῖοι.

26. "A nosebleed is congenial to all inflamed internal tumors": Cf. Galen, *De crisibus* 3.3 (ed. Kühn, 9:708; ed. Alexanderson, 170 lines 15–16): πάσας δὲ ... τὰς φλεγμονὰς ... ἡ διὰ ῥινῶν αἱμορραγία κρίνει (all inflamed tumors ... are brought to a crisis through a nosebleed).

27. Galen, *De crisibus* 3.3 (ed. Kühn, 9:708; ed. Alexanderson, 170–71); cf. R. Moshe Narboni, *Sefer Oraḥ Ḥayyim* (MS Munich 276, fol. 133b).

28. "tumors . . . at the roots of the ears": Cf. Galen, *De crisibus* 3.3 (ed. Kühn, 9:709; ed. Alexanderson, 171 line 10): παρωτίδες (tumors of the parotid glands).

29. "tumors and abscesses": Cf. Galen, *De crisibus* 3.3 (ed. Kühn, 9:709; ed. Alexanderson, 171 line 11): ἀποσκήμματα (determination of humors to one part of the body). The translator has obviously read the Greek ἀποσκήμματα as ἀποστήματα.

30. Galen, *De crisibus* 3.3 (ed. Kühn, 9:709; ed. Alexanderson, 171 lines 10–13); cf. R. Moshe Narboni, *Sefer Oraḥ Ḥayyim* (MS Munich 276, fol. 133b).

31. "especially since a crisis may occur that does not necessarily follow from such signs": Cf. Galen, *De crisibus* 3.10 (ed. Kühn, 9:7511; ed. Alexanderson, 199 lines 4–5): καὶ μᾶλλον ὅταν ἄσημοι τυγχάνωσι γινόμεναι (and especially since these crises sometimes come without [prognostic] signs).

32. "reliable and accurate": Cf. Galen, *De crisibus* 3.10 (ed. Kühn, 9:751; ed. Alexanderson, 199 line 3): ἀκριβεῖς.

33. Galen, *De crisibus* 3.10 (ed. Kühn, 9:751; ed. Alexanderson, 199 lines 3–6).

34. Galen, *De diebus decretoriis* 1.6 (ed. Kühn, 9:796–97).

35. Galen, *De diebus decretoriis* 1.4 (ed. Kühn, 9:784).

36. "closest": Cf. Galen, *De diebus decretoriis* 1.5 (ed. Kühn, 9:792): μάλιστα μιμεῖται.

37. "are close to the nature of the fourteenth": Cf. Galen, *De diebus decretoriis* 1.5 (ed. Kühn, 9:792): πλήσιον δ᾽ αὐτῶν ("are close to these"—i.e., to the fourteenth and the seventh day).

38. "Next [in closeness] comes the fourth day, and then the third, fifth, and eighteenth": Cf. Galen, *De diebus decretoriis* 1.5 (ed. Kühn, 9:792): "Next in closeness are the seventeenth and fifth day, and then the fourth and then the third and the eighteenth [day]" (trans. Gerrit Bos).

39. Galen, *De diebus decretoriis* 1.5 (ed. Kühn, 9:792).

40. "critical movement is weaker in all of them and slowly becomes less": Cf. Galen, *De diebus decretoriis* 1.10 (ed. Kühn, 9:817): ἐκλύουσι κατὰ βραχυ τὸ ἀγωνιστικόν.

41. Galen, *De diebus decretoriis* 1.10 (ed. Kühn, 9:817).

42. Galen, *De diebus decretoriis* 1.2 (ed. Kühn, 9:774–75).

43. Galen, *De diebus decretoriis* 1.5 (ed. Kühn, 9:792).

44. "not a true one": Cf. Galen, *De diebus decretoriis* 1.2 (ed. Kühn, 9:776): ἄπιστον.

45. "without previous announcement": I.e., without prognostic signs.

46. Galen, *De diebus decretoriis* 1.2 (ed. Kühn, 9:776).

47. "very acute to the extreme": Cf. Galen, *De diebus decretoriis* 2.12 (ed. Kühn, 9:886): ἀκριβῶς . . . κάτοξυ.

48. "absolutely acute": Cf. Galen, *De diebus decretoriis* 2.12 (ed. Kühn, 9:886): ἀκριβῶς . . . ὀξὺ.

49. The text does not feature in Galen, *De diebus decretoriis* 1, but in *De diebus decretoriis* 2.12 (ed. Kühn, 9:886).

50. "from the nature of the illness, as is . . . culminations": Cf. Galen, *De crisibus* 1.4 (ed. Kühn, 9:561); cf. Maimonides, *Aphorisms* 25.45 (ed. and trans. Bos, forthcoming).

51. Galen, *De crisibus* 1.4 (ed. Kühn, 9:561–63).

52. Galen, *In Hippocratis Epidemiarum* 2.1 (ed. Wenkebach and Pfaff [CMG 5.10.1], 177 lines 35–42).

53. By inclusive reckoning.

54. Galen, *In Hippocratis Epidemiarum* 2.6 (ed. Wenkebach and Pfaff [CMG 5.10.1], 370 lines 30–42).

55. Galen, *In Hippocratis Aphorismos commentarius* 4.36 (ed. Kühn, 17B:712).

56. Galen, *In Hippocratis Prognostica commentarius* 3.7 (ed. Kühn, 18B:246).

57. "From . . . relaxation": Cf. Maimonides, *Commentary on Hippocrates' Aphorisms* 1.20 (ed. Bos): "Galen says that a complete crisis is a combination of six things. The first is that the humors must be cocted. The second is that this occurs on one of the days of the crisis. The third is that [the crisis] occurs with plain matter that is evacuated from the body, but not with an abscess. The fourth is that the evacuated matter only consists of the harmful matter that causes the illness. The fifth is that the evacuation is from the same side as the illness. The sixth is that it is accompanied by relaxation and lightness of the body. Says Galen: If one or more of these [conditions] are missing, the crisis is neither perfect nor complete."

58. Galen, *In Hippocratis Aphorismos commentarius* 1.20 (ed. Kühn, 17B:438), only mentions five indications, since he combines the first and the fifth one as follows: "The fifth is that it (i.e., the evacuation) is done on a critical day when there is coction [of superfluous matter]."

59. Galen, *In Hippocratis Aphorismos commentarius* 1.20 (ed. Kühn, 17B:438); cf. Anastassiou and Irmer, eds., *Testimonien zum Corpus Hippocraticum*, 1:463.

The Twelfth Treatise

1. Galen, *De curandi ratione per venae sectionem* 9 (ed. Kühn, 11:278–79; trans. Brain, 81).

2. Galen, *De curandi ratione per venae sectionem* 13 (ed. Kühn, 11:290; trans. Brain, 87).

3. "the external condition [of the body]": Cf. Galen, *De curandi ratione per venae sectionem* 13 (ed. Kühn, 11:291): ἕξις (condition).

4. "even if their blood is like that of those who are in the prime of their life": Cf. Galen, *De curandi ratione per venae sectionem* 13 (ed. Kühn, 11:291): εἰ καὶ τὴν αὐτὴν ἔχειν φαίνονται διάθεσιν ἀκμαστικῷ σώματι.

5. Galen, *De curandi ratione per venae sectionem* 13 (ed. Kühn, 11:291; trans. Brain, 87).

6. Galen, *De curandi ratione per venae sectionem* 19 (ed. Kühn, 11:308; trans. Brain, 95).

7. "flabby": Cf. Galen, *Ad Glauconem de medendi methodo* 1.15 (ed. Kühn, 11:46): βρυώδης.

8. Galen, *Ad Glauconem de medendi methodo* 1.15 (ed. Kühn, 11:43–46).

9. "animal faculty": I.e., vital faculty. The Greek term ζωτικός, esp. in combination with πνεῦμα, has become in Arabic, as a result of a wrong translation, *ḥayawānī* (animal); see Ullmann, *Islamic Medicine*, 63.

10. Galen, *De curandi ratione per venae sectionem* 6 (ed. Kühn, 11:269; trans. Brain, 76).

11. "[venesection should not be applied]": Cf. Galen, *De sanitate tuenda* 4.5 (ed. Koch [CMG 5.4.2], 116 line 7): μήτε φλεβοτομεῖν.

12. "in a [significant] quantity": Cf. Galen, *De sanitate tuenda* 4.5 (ed. Koch [CMG 5.4.2], 116 line 12): ἀξιολόγως (worth mentioning).

13. Galen, *De sanitate tuenda* 4.5 (ed. Koch [CMG 5.4.2], 116 lines 5–25).

14. I.e., putting him on a diet.

15. "fullness": "tolerance" (**ELU**).

16. Galen, *De methodo medendi* 4.6 (ed. Kühn, 10:287–88). Cf. Maimonides, *On Asthma* 13.32 (ed. and trans. Bos, 1:99).

17. Galen, *De methodo medendi* 5.14 (ed. Kühn, 10:375).

18. Galen, *De methodo medendi* 9.5 (ed. Kühn, 10:625).

19. Galen, *De methodo medendi* 9.5 (ed. Kühn, 10:624–25).

20. "of the ankle": Cf. Galen, *In Hippocratis Aphorismos commentarius* 2.17 (ed. Kühn, 17B:482): τῶν σφυρῶν. All the manuscripts have the faulty reading "of the neck," resulting from a corruption of the Arabic *al-kāḥil* (ankle) as *al-kāhil* (neck).

21. Galen, *In Hippocratis Aphorismos commentarius* 2.17 (ed. Kühn, 17B:481–82).

22. "major": Lit., precious.

23. Galen, *De curandi ratione per venae sectionem* 12 (ed. Kühn, 11:287; trans. Brain, 85–86).

24. "animal": I.e., vital; cf. aphorism 12.5, above.

25. Galen, *De curandi ratione per venae sectionem* 5 (ed. Kühn, 11:265, 269; trans. Brain, 85–86).

26. "I know . . . fever": Cf. Galen, *De curandi ratione per venae sectionem* 12 (ed. Kühn, 11:287): ὥστε ἐνίων οἶδα κοτύλας ἓξ ἀφελεῖν εὐθέως ἤτοι κατὰ τὴν δευτέραν ἢ τὴν τρίτην ἢ τὴν τετάρτην ἡμέραν. Trans. Brain, 85: "I know, for instance, of some doctors who take six *cotyles* (note: about 1,700 ml) either all at once or spread over two, three or four days." Brain interpreted the Greek ἐνίων as referring to some doctors, instead of to some of Galen's own patients; see as well ibid. (ed. Kühn, 11:294; trans. Brain, 89): "I have known myself to remove as much as six pounds of blood from some patients." Brain misinterpreted the Greek εὐθέως ἤτοι κατὰ τὴν δευτέραν ἢ τὴν τρίτην ἢ τὴν τετάρτην ἡμέραν. The weight of the *raṭl* varies according to region and period; see Hinz, *Islamische Masse*, 28–33.

27. Galen, *De curandi ratione per venae sectionem* 12 (ed. Kühn, 11:287, 294; trans. Brain, 85, 89).

28. Galen, *De curandi ratione per venae sectionem* 12 (ed. Kühn, 11:286–87; trans. Brain, 85).

29. I.e., draw all the blood on that very same day.

30. I.e., to divert the blood from a diseased region in one part of the body to another. The sentence "But . . . direction" is missing in ed. Kühn, 11:311–12,

but features in trans. Brain, 97 n. 86, following MS Florence, Laurentiana Plut. 74.22 (see Brain, p. xii): ἐφ ὧν δε ἀντισπασεται (but for those who are revulsed [trans. Brain, 97]).

31. "it is better to repeat it [i.e., to do so] on the second and third day": Cf. Galen, *De curandi ratione per venae sectionem* 21 (ed. Kühn, 11:312): κἂν δύο ταῖς ἐφεξῆς ἡμέραις γένηται, βέλτιον ἐστί; ibid. (trans. Brain, 97): "it is better that it should be done on two successive days."

32. Galen, *De curandi ratione per venae sectionem* 21 (ed. Kühn, 11:311–12; trans. Brain, 97).

33. "to a reduction in the intensity of the flow": Cf. Galen, *De curandi ratione per venae sectionem* 14 (ed. Kühn, 11:292): τῷ τόνῳ δὲ τῆς ῥύσεως ὀκλάζοντι.

34. "change": Cf. Galen, *De curandi ratione per venae sectionem* 14 (ed. Kühn, 11:292): μεταβολή.

35. "But a change toward weakness is something I do not have to discuss": Cf. Galen, *De curandi ratione per venae sectionem* 14 (ed. Kühn, 11:292; trans. Brain, 88): "What more is there to say about the change towards indistinctness, since you have learned that in this quality there is a sound criterion of the strength, as well as the weakness, of the faculties?"

36. Galen, *De curandi ratione per venae sectionem* 14 (ed. Kühn, 11:291–92; trans. Brain, 88).

37. Galen, *De curandi ratione per venae sectionem* 16 (ed. Kühn, 11:297; trans. Brain, 90).

38. Galen, *De methodo medendi* 4.6 (ed. Kühn, 10:287–88).

39. "the impossiblity of dissolution": Cf. Galen, *De methodo medendi* 9.10 (ed. Kühn, 10:639): στέγνωσις; supplement to Ullmann, *Wörterbuch zu den griechisch-arabischen,* 2:329.

40. Galen, *De methodo medendi* 9.10 (ed. Kühn, 10:639).

41. Galen, *De curandi ratione per venae sectionem* 7 (ed. Kühn, 11:270–73; trans. Brain, 77–78).

42. "ulcerous fatigue": Galen's following discussion concerns "inflammatory" fatigue (φλεγμονώδη); cf. Galen, *De sanitate tuenda* 4.10 (ed. Koch [CMG 5.4.2], 131 line 2).

43. I.e., the physician.

44. Galen, *De sanitate tuenda* 4.10 (ed. Koch [CMG 5.4.2], 131 lines 2, 10–11, 19–25).

45. "on the spine": Lit., to the spine.

46. Galen, *De methodo medendi* 6.3; ed. Kühn, 10:406–7.

47. Galen, *De curandi ratione per venae sectionem* 20–21 (ed. Kühn, 11:309–11; trans. Brain, 96–97).

48. "when you find that the patient is fit for bleeding": Cf. Galen, *De curandi ratione per venae sectionem* 20 (ed. Kühn, 11:309–10): ἐν ᾗ γὰρ ἂν ἡμέρᾳ τοὺς σκοποὺς τῆς φλεβοτομίας ἐπὶ τοῦ κάμνοντος εὑρίσκῃς; ibid. (trans. Brain, 96): "For on whatever day you observe the indications for phlebotomy in the patient."

49. Galen, *De curandi ratione per venae sectionem* 20 (ed. Kühn, 11:309–10; trans. Brain, 96).

50. Galen, *De anatomia magna* 3.6 (ed. Kühn, 2:388).
51. Galen, *In Hippocratis Epidemiarum* 6.1 (ed. Wenkebach and Pfaff [CMG 5.10.2.2], 28 lines 3–5; Deller translation, 532, no. 61).
52. "at the inner side of the knee ": Cf. Galen, *De curandi ratione per venae sectionem* 18 (ed. Kühn, 11:302): ἐπ' ἰγνύων (at the hams).
53. "at the inner side of the arm": Cf. Galen, *De curandi ratione per venae sectionem* 18 (ed. Kühn, 11:303): ἐπ' ἀγκῶνος (at the elbow); i.e., the cubital vein.
54. Galen, *De curandi ratione per venae sectionem* 16.18 (ed. Kühn, 11:298, 302–3; trans. Brain, 90, 93).
55. Galen, *De compositione medicamentorum secundum locos* 10.2 (ed. Kühn, 13:335). For the Arabic *mayāmir*, coined after the Syriac *mēmrā*, see Ullmann, *Medizin im Islam*, 48, no. 50.
56. "from the one at the inner side of the knee": Cf. Galen, *De curandi ratione per venae sectionem* 18 (ed. Kühn, 11:305): ἀπὸ τῆς ἰγνύος (from the ham).
57. "As for . . . patients": Cf. Galen, *De curandi ratione per venae sectionem* 18 (ed. Kühn, 11:304–5; trans. Brain, 93–94): "I have known diseases of the hip cured in one day by an evacuation through the legs; such of them, that is, as have not arisen as a result of cold, but through blood having collected in the veins in the ischial region. Hence phlebotomy from the ham is more effective than from the ankles in patients thus affected, and scarification brings them no obvious benefit."
58. Galen, *De curandi ratione per venae sectionem* 18 (ed. Kühn, 11:304–5; trans. Brain, 93–94).
59. I.e., those in the legs.
60. Galen, *De curandi ratione per venae sectionem* 19 (ed. Kühn, 11:307–8; trans. Brain, 94–95).
61. "When an [inflamed] tumor starts to develop in the parts of the mouth": Cf. Galen, *De methodo medendi* 13.11 (ed. Kühn, 10:904): ἐπὶ δὲ συνάγχης (in the case of angina).
62. Galen, *De methodo medendi* 13.11 (ed. Kühn, 10:904).
63. "When the illness is in the neck": Cf. Galen, *De methodo medendi* 13.11 (ed. Kühn, 10:904): τῶν δὲ κατ' ἰνίον πασχόντων (for those affected in the region of the occiput).
64. "namely, the saphenous": Added by Maimonides.
65. Galen, *De methodo medendi* 13.11 (ed. Kühn, 10:904).
66. "the basilic vein": Added by Maimonides; cf. Galen, *De curandi ratione per venae sectionem* 16 (ed. Kühn, 11:297).
67. Galen, *De curandi ratione per venae sectionem* 16 (ed. Kühn, 11:296–97; trans. Brain, 90).
68. "on the same side as": Lit., parallel to; cf. Galen, *De curandi ratione per venae sectionem* 16 (ed. Kühn, 11:297): κατ'εὐθύ.
69. "sometimes": Cf. Galen, *De curandi ratione per venae sectionem* 16 (ed. Kühn, 11:297): πολλάκις (often).
70. Galen, *De curandi ratione per venae sectionem* 16 (ed. Kühn, 11:297; trans. Brain, 90).
71. Galen, *De methodo medendi* 5.6 (ed. Kühn, 10:331–32).

72. "membranes": Presumably the peritoneum and pleura. Galen, *De curandi ratione per venae sectionem* 23 (ed. Kühn, 11:316; trans. Brain, 98 n. 92).

73. "aneurysm" (*umm al-dam?*): Cf. Galen, *De curandi ratione per venae sectionem* 23 (ed. Kühn, 11:313): ἀνεύρυσμα.

74. Galen, *De curandi ratione per venae sectionem* 22–23 (ed. Kühn, 11:312–16; trans. Brain, 97–99).

75. Galen, *In Hippocratis Epidemiarum* 6.1 (ed. Wenkebach and Pfaff [CMG 5.10.2.2], 27 line 28–28 line 3; Deller translation, 532, no. 60).

76. "This is a most important diagnostic rule": Not in Galen, *De locis affectis* 3 (ed. Kühn, 8:185).

77. Galen, *De locis affectis* 3 (ed. Kühn, 8:185).

78. "pure red": Cf. Galen, *Ad Glauconem de methodo medendi* 1.12 (ed. Kühn, 11:38): ξανθός (reddish yellow).

79. Galen, *Ad Glauconem de methodo medendi* 1.12 (ed. Kühn, 11:37–38).

80. Galen, *In Hippocratis Epidemiarum* 6.7 (ed. Wenkebach and Pfaff [CMG 5.10.2.2], 421 lines 13–20; Deller translation, 542, no. 109).

81. "the hollow in the back of the neck" (*nuqra*): Cf. Lane, *Arabic-English Lexicon*, 2838: "The place where the occiput ends at, in the back part of the neck; i.e., the hollow in the back of the neck;" cf. Galen, *In Hippocratis De humoribus commentarius* 1.14 (ed. Kühn, 16:150): ἰνίον.

82. "to attract . . . [in the opposite direction]": Cf. Galen, *In Hippocratis De humoribus commentarius* 1.14 (ed. Kühn, 16:150): ὡς ἀντισπᾶσθαι.

83. See introduction.

84. Galen, *De curandi ratione per venae sectionem* 10 (ed. Kühn, 11:282; trans. Brain, 83).

85. Galen, *De compositione medicamentorum secundum locos* 9.2 (ed. Kühn, 13:256).

86. Galen, *De methodo medendi*, 10.17–18 (ed. Kühn, 10:798).

87. "diversion": Lit., evacuation of the blood through diversion; cf. Galen, *De methodo medendi* 12.8 (ed. Kühn, 10:861): παροχευτέον.

88. Galen, *De methodo medendi* 12.8 (ed. Kühn, 10:861).

The Thirteenth Treatise

1. Galen, *In Hippocratis De acutorum morborum victu et Galeni commentarius* 2.11 (ed. Helmreich [CMG 5.9.1], 173 lines 19–21).

2. "Compound purgatives are bad": Cf. Galen, *In Hippocratis de acutorum morborum victu et Galeni commentarius* 2.11 (ed. Helmreich [CMG 5.9.1], 173 line 25): ἡ γὰρ στάσις ἐν ταῖς μίξεσι τῶν καθαιρόντων γίνεται φαρμάκων (for discord occurs in compound purgatives).

3. Galen, *In Hippocratis de acutorum morborum victu et Galeni commentarius* 2.11 (ed. Helmreich [CMG 5.9.1], 173 lines 25–29).

4. For its seven varieties, see Maimonides, *Glossary of Drug Names*, ed. Rosner, no. 178.

5. Galen, *In Hippocratis De acutorum morborum victu et Galeni commentarius* 2.12 (ed. Helmreich [CMG 5.9.1], 173 lines 20–24).

6. I.e., after taking purgatives.

7. Galen, *In Hippocratis De acutorum morborum victu et Galeni commentarius* 2.12 (ed. Helmreich [CMG 5.9.1], 175 lines 24–29).

8. "myrtle" (*rayḥān*): Instead of myrtle, it is possible that Maimonides meant basil (*Ocimum basilicum*), for while the term *rayḥān* (lit., "fragrant") was used to refer to myrtle in the Maghreb, basil was used in the East. Cf. Maimonides, *Glossary of Drug Names*, ed. Rosner, no. 10; Dioscurides, *Dioscurides Triumphans*, 2.124 (ed. Dietrich).

9. Galen, *In Hippocratis Aphorismos commentarius* 3.15 (ed. Kühn, 17B:600–601).

10. "a number of times": Lit., a number of successive times.

11. "If you want to purge [the body], first use a laxative for a number of times; and if you want to apply emesis, first stimulate [the body] repeatedly": Cf. Galen, *In Hippocratis Aphorismos commentarius* 2.9 (ed. Kühn, 17B:464): "Most people want the bodies of those who are to be purged to be made loose, whether they are going to be purged with emetic drugs through irritation with emetics or through drugs that purge downwards through frequently emptying the gut." I.e., the body should be made loose (pores opened, blockages removed) before the application of the specific purgatives, whether they purge by emesis or vacuation, hence they think it right to prepare the body first before actually giving the purgative. The Greek as it stands is impossible, and ed. Kühn's Latin translation, although better, still presents problems.

12. Galen, *In Hippocratis Aphorismos commentarius* 2.9 (ed. Kühn, 17B:464–66).

13. Galen, *De methodo medendi* 14.16 (ed. Kühn, 10:1010).

14. Galen, *De sanitate tuenda* 4.5 (ed. Koch [CMG 5.4.2], 116 lines 12–17; trans. Green, 160).

15. I could not identify this quotation.

16. Galen, *De sanitate tuenda* 6.13 (ed. Koch [CMG 5.4.2], 194 lines 19–23).

17. "If, at the end of the treatment, one needs drugs to expel the black bile, use these": Cf. Galen, *De methodo medendi* 5.14: ὕστερον δ' ἂν, εἰ δεήσει, καὶ τοῖς τὰ μέλανα καθαίρουσι χρήσαιο (At the end, if necessary, one may also use those drugs that purge the black bile).

18. Galen, *De methodo medendi* 5.14.

19. Galen, *De simplicium medicamentorum temperamentis ac facultatibus* 3.28 (ed. Kühn, 11:617–18).

20. Galen, *De simplicium medicamentorum temperamentis ac facultatibus* 3.27 (ed. Kühn, 11:616).

21. Galen, *De simplicium medicamentorum temperamentis ac facultatibus* 3.27 (ed. Kühn, 11:615).

22. Galen, *De simplicium medicamentorum temperamentis ac facultatibus* 3.26 (ed. Kühn, 11:614–15).

23. "remedies": Cf. Galen, *De optimo medico cognoscendo* 11.8 (Arabic translation Ḥunayn, ed. and trans. Iskandar, 122 line 13): "fruit."

24. This treatise has been lost in the original Greek. For the Arabic translation, see Iskandar, ed. and trans., 122 lines 10–13.

25. Galen, *In Hippocratis Epidemiarum* 6.5 (ed. Wenkebach and Pfaff [CMG 5.10.2.2], 310 line 1ff; Deller translation, 539, no. 94).

26. The closest parallel I could find in *In Hippocratis De humoribus commentarius* 1.12 (ed. Kühn, 16:125) is "Just as we administer an evacuating drug, when melancholic humors are abundant in the case of melancholy, cancer, and elephantiasis, in the same way we use drugs to purge the phlegm in the case of epilepsy." Cf. Deichgräber, *Hippokrates' De humoribus,* 48; and aphorism 12.43 above.

27. Galen, *In Hippocratis Epidemiarum* 2.3 (ed. Wenkebach and Pfaff [CMG 5.10.1], 264 lines 32–35; Deller translation, 525, no. 25); cf. Anastassiou and Irmer, *Testimonien zum Corpus Hippocraticum,* 1:218 (trans. Littré, 5:104 lines 4–5).

28. "is disordered in his regimen": Cf. Galen, *De curandi ratione per venae sectionem* 10 (ed. Kühn, 11:272; trans. Brain, 83): γαστριμάργους (gluttonous).

29. Galen, *De curandi ratione per venae sectionem* 10 (ed. Kühn, 11:272; trans. Brain, 77).

30. "just like that": Lit., interrupted.

31. Galen, *In Hippocratis Epidemiarum* 2.1 (ed. Wenkebach and Pfaff [CMG 5.10.1], 201 lines 5–9; Deller translation, 524, no. 19).

32. "shreds": That is, of intestinal tissue. Cf. Galen, *In Hippocratis Epidemiarum* 2.1 (ed. Wenkebach and Pfaff [CMG 5.10.1], 199 line 39): "Durchfall" (diarrhea).

33. The text is corrupt; my translation follows **NB**.

34. Not in Galen, *In Hippocratis Epidemiarum* 2.1 (ed. Wenkebach and Pfaff [CMG 5.10.1]).

35. Galen, *In Hippocratis Epidemiarum* 2.1 (ed. Wenkebach and Pfaff [CMG 5.10.1], 199 line 35–200 line 1; not in Deller translation).

36. Galen, *In Hippocratis De acutorum morborum victu et Galeni commentarius* 2.12 (ed. Helmreich [CMG 5.9.1], 174 lines 18–20, 27–29).

37. Galen, *In Hippocratis De acutorum morborum victu et Galeni commentarius* 2.13 (ed. Helmreich [CMG 5.9.1], 176 lines 15–19).

38. Galen, *In Hippocratis De acutorum morborum victu et Galeni commentarius* 2.11, (ed. Helmreich [CMG 5.9.1], 174 lines 11–13).

39. "in the liver or in another organ": The Hippocratic text speaks of an abscess (ἀπόστημα) in the flank (κενέων) while the Galenic text as preserved in the Arabic tradition speaks of an abscess in the region of the flank. Cf. Galen, *In Hippocratis Epidemiarum* 2.2 (ed. Wenkebach and Pfaff [CMG 5.10.1], 200 line 32; 201 line 2).

40. Galen, *In Hippocratis Epidemiarum* 2.2 (ed. Wenkebach and Pfaff [CMG 5.10.1], 201 lines 5–9; Deller translation, 524, no. 20).

41. "especially" (*bi-kathra*): Cf. Oribasius, *Collectiones Medicae* 7.23 (ed. Raeder [CMG 6.1], 224 line 12): μάλιστα. See also Deichgräber, *Hippokrates' De humoribus,* 46.

42. Galen, *In Hippocratis De humoribus commentarius* 2.13 (ed. Kühn, 16:255).

43. Galen, *De optimo medico cognoscendo* 11.8 (Arabic translation Ḥunayn, ed. and trans. Iskandar, 122 lines 14–16).

44. Galen, *De sanitate tuenda* 5.9 (ed. Kühn, 6:356).

45. Galen, *In Hippocratis Epidemiarum* 6.5 (ed. Wenkebach and Pfaff [CMG 5.10.2.2], 316 line 23–317 line 9; Deller translation, 539–40, no. 45).

46. I could not locate this quotation in book 3 of *In Hippocratis De acutorum morborum victu et Galeni commentarius.* However, in 1.44 (ed. Helmreich [CMG 5.9.1], 160 lines 15–18) Hippocrates remarks in the context of someone suffering from fever: "If the previous food which the patient has recently eaten should not have gone down, give an enema if the patient be strong and in the prime of life, but if he be too weak use a suppository, should the bowels be not well moved of their own accord" (Hippocrates, *Regimen in Acute Diseases,* trans. Jones, 79).

47. For this pseudo-Galenic treatise, cf. aphorism 10.52 above.

48. Galen, *In Hippocratis Epidemiarum* 6.6 (ed. Wenkebach and Pfaff [CMG 5.10.2.2], 340 lines 7–11; Deller translation, 540, no. 100).

49. "scales" (*qushūr*): Cf. Pseudo-Galen, *In Hippocratis De humoribus commentarius* 1.12 (ed. Kühn, 16:147): λεπίδας. Also cf. Liddell-Scott, *Greek-English Lexicon,* 1039: "epithelial debris; scales"; supplement to Ullmann, *Wörterbuch zu den griechisch-arabischen,* 1:623. Epithelial debris means the debris of the epithelium, the cellular covering of the mucous membranes.

50. "putrefaction": Cf. Pseudo-Galen, *In Hippocratis De humoribus commentarius* 1.12 (ed. Kühn, 16:147): περιττώμα (superfluity).

51. Psuedo-Galen, *In Hippocratis De humoribus commentarius* 1.12 (ed. Kühn, 16:146–47).

52. "the other types of evacuation": i.e., except for those mentioned before—evacuations that one applies in the case of patients who do not eat much and who are used to being evacuated. Cf. Galen, *Ad Glauconem de methodo medendi* 1.15 (ed. Kühn, 11:45).

53. Galen, *Ad Glauconem de methodo medendi* 1.15 (ed. Kühn, 11:46).

54. Galen, *De simplicium medicamentorum temperamentis ac facultatibus* 10.8 (ed. Kühn, 12:267–68).

55. Galen, *De sanitate tuenda* 5.9 (ed. Kühn, 6:356).

56. Galen, *De methodo medendi* 11.15 (ed. Kühn, 10:781).

57. Galen, *De methodo medendi* 12.8 (ed. Kühn, 10:871).

58. Galen, *De compositione medicamentorum secundum locos* 9.5 (ed. Kühn, 13:295–96). Maimonides has turned Galen's concrete recipe, which gives only the concrete ingredients with their weights, into a more general abstract prescription covering all the ingredients with the mentioned properties.

59. Cf. Maimonides and Gerrit Bos in Maimonides, *On Asthma,* Author's Introduction (1:4, esp. n. 13), 13.0 (1:80, esp. n. 2).

60. These *waṣāyā* are possibly part of a lost composition by Abū al-ʿAlāʾ ibn Zuhr (d. 525 AH/1131 AD) known as the *Waṣiya* in a quotation by Ibn al-Muṭrān (see Ullmann, *Medizin im Islam,* 162; Álvarez Millán, *Actualización del corpus médico-literario de los Banū Zuhr,* 178); for his literary activity see Ullmann, *Medizin im Islam,* 162–63; Álvarez Millán, ibid.

61. See Maimonides, *On Asthma* 9.1 (ed. and trans. Bos, 1:40); Ullmann, *Medizin im Islam,* 162–63; Álvarez Millán, *Actualización del corpus médico-literario de los Banū Zuhr,* 178.

62. "rob": I.e., inspissated juice.

63. I.e., relieves the bowels.

64. I.e., what he stated above (aphorism 13.49)—that these purgatives should not be mixed with musk or wine.

65. On al-Tamīmī (d. 370/980) and his *Kitāb al-murshid fī jawāhir al-aghdhiya wa-quwāt al-mufradāt min al-adwiya* (Guide to the substances of foodstuffs and the powers of simple drugs) see Ullmann, *Medizin im Islam,* 269–70; Schönfeld, "Das 14. Kapitel aus dem *Kitāb al-Muršid.*"

The Fourteenth Treatise

1. Galen, *De usu partium* 5.4 (ed. Helmreich 1:262–63; trans. May 1:253–54).

2. Galen, *De sanitate tuenda* 4.6 (ed. Koch [CMG 5.4.2], 122 line 33–123 line 1), speaks about someone who suffers from fatigue and whose veins are full of unconcocted humors.

3. Galen, *De sanitate tuenda* 4.6 (ed. Koch [CMG 5.4.2], 122 line 33–123 line 13).

4. I could not locate this text in Pseudo-Galen's *In Hippocratis De humoribus commentarius* 1 (ed. Kühn, 16:1–207).

5. Galen, *In Hippocratis Aphorismos commentarius* 4.12 (ed. Kühn, 17B:671).

6. "not to induce vomiting, but to soften the stool": Cf. Galen, *Ad Glauconem de methodo medendi* 1.15 (ed. Kühn, 11:55): "not only to induce vomiting, but also to soften the stool."

7. Galen, *Ad Glauconem de methodo medendi* 1.15 (ed. Kühn, 11:55).

8. Galen, *De sanitate tuenda* 6.3 (ed. Koch [CMG 5.4.2], 172 lines 15–17, 29–31).

9. Galen, *De methodo medendi* 6.11 (ed. Kühn, 10:517).

10. Galen, *De alimentorum facultatibus* 3.8 (ed. Kühn, 6:677).

11. Galen, *In Hippocratis Epidemiarum* 2.6 (ed. Wenkebach and Pfaff [CMG 5.10.1], 407 lines 35–40; Deller translation, 528, no. 40).

12. Galen's commentary on Hippocrates' *Diseases of Women* is of doubtful authenticity (cf. the introduction to this volume, pp. xv–xvi). However, this quotation is certainly inauthentic since its subject bears no relation to that of women's diseases; such a collection of unrelated and thus inauthentic prescriptions is already found in the Hippocratic text itself: Littré, trans., *Oeuvres complètes d'Hippocrate,* 1:92–109). See also Ullmann, *Zwei spätantike Kommentare,* 245.

13. Galen, *In Hippocratis De natura hominis commentarius* 3.22 (ed. Mewaldt, 105); the text is probably corrupt. In his commentary on Hippocrates' *Regimen of Health* 5 (trans. Jones, 53): "He who is in the habit of taking an emetic twice a month will find it better to do on two successive days than once every fortnight," Galen states that this text needs elucidation because Hippocrates has not made any distinction about those who vomit twice a month, and then continues: "For some I think that it is good to vomit [twice a month] in order to empty [the body] . . . But for others [it is good] in order to cleanse the thick, viscous humor which has settled in the stomach. In both cases nothing hinders them from doing so when there is an interval, but not so when one does so on two consecutive days."

14. Galen, *De methodo medendi* 12.8 (ed. Kühn, 10:871).
15. Galen, *In Hippocratis Aphorismos commentarius* 4.14 (ed. Kühn, 17B:674).
16. Galen, *In Hippocratis De natura hominis commentarius* 3.18 (ed. Mewaldt, 102 lines 7–9).

The Fifteenth Treatise

1. Galen, *De compositione medicamentorum per genera* 5.14 (ed. Kühn, 13:851–52); for the title *Qāṭājānas* (κατά γενός), cf. Steinschneider, *Griechischen Ärzte*, 291 (343).
2. Galen, *De compositione medicamentorum per genera* 5.15 (ed. Kühn, 13:851–55).
3. Cf. **C**: "One should also refrain from cauterization in the case of bodily parts that have depth, especially when the part has a deep hollowness, for all the parts have hollowness except the hands, feet, and thighs." This quotation does not feature in the Hebrew translation edited by Wasserstein; cf. Maimonides, *Medical Aphorisms* 25.18 (ed. and trans. Bos, forthcoming); and the introduction to this volume (pp. xix–xx).
4. Galen, *In Hippocratis Aphorismos commentarius* 6.27 (ed. Kühn18A:39); Anastassiou and Irmer, *Testimonien zum Corpus Hippocraticum*, 1:314 (trans. Littré, 7:166 line 2); cf. Maimonides, *Medical Aphorisms* 25.18 (ed. and trans. Bos, forthcoming); and the introduction to this volume (pp. xix–xx).
5. Galen, *In Hippocratis Epidemiarum* 6.6, (ed. Wenkebach and Pfaff [CMG 5.10.2.2], 338 lines 6–9; Deller translation, 540, no. 99). Guy de Chauliac possibly refers to the Latin translation of this text in his *Inventarium sive Chirurgia Magna*, 1:230 lines 1–2; 2.188.
6. Galen, *In Hippocratis Epidemiarum* 6.6 (ed. Wenkebach and Pfaff [CMG 5.10.2.2], 421 lines 35–40; Deller translation, 542, no. 109); cf. Maimonides, *Medical Aphorisms* 25.18 (ed. and trans. Bos, forthcoming); and the introduction to this volume (pp. xix–xx).
7. Galen, *Ad Glauconem de methodo medendi* 2.2 (ed. Kühn, 11:83).
8. "[more than any other]": Cf. Galen, *Ad Glauconem de methodo medendi* 2.3 (ed. Kühn, 11:88): μάλιστα.
9. Galen, *Ad Glauconem de methodo medendi* 2.3 (ed. Kühn, 11:88).
10. Galen, *Ad Glauconem de methodo medendi* 2.11 (ed. Kühn, 11:135–36).
11. "bitter vetch . . . with vinegar and darnel . . . flour with honey": Cf. Galen, *Ad Glauconem de methodo medendi* 2.11 (ed. Kühn, 11:136): "oxymel with bitter vetch or with darnel flour."
12. Galen, *Ad Glauconem de methodo medendi* 2.11 (ed. Kühn, 11:136).
13. "pudenda": Cf. Galen, *Ad Glauconem de methodo medendi* 2.11 (ed. Kühn, 11:137): αἰδοία; supplement to Ullmann, *Wörterbuch zu den griechisch-arabischen*, 1:72.
14. Galen, *Ad Glauconem de methodo medendi* 2.11 (ed. Kühn, 11:137).
15. Galen, *Ad Glauconem de methodo medendi* '2.12 (ed. Kühn, 11:141).
16. "a headache affecting the whole head" (*khūdha*; i.e., helmet): Cf. Thies, *Erkrankungen des Gehirns*, 40–41; supplement to Ullmann, *Wörterbuch zu den griechisch-arabischen*, 1:550, s.v. κεφαλαία.
17. Galen, *De locis affectis* 3.12 (ed. Kühn, 8:202–3).

18. Galen, *De methodo medendi* 4.6 (ed. Kühn, 10:290).
19. Galen, *De methodo medendi* 4.7 (ed. Kühn, 10:296).
20. I.e., making the wound larger.
21. Galen, *De methodo medendi* 6.2 (ed. Kühn, 10:391–92).
22. Cf. Galen, *De methodo medendi* 14.9 (ed. Kühn, 10:979): εἶτα θεράπευε τοῖς ἄλλοις ἕλκεσι παραπλησίως.
23. Galen, *De methodo medendi* 14.9 (ed. Kühn, 10:979).
24. I.e., glands.
25. Galen, *De methodo medendi* 14.9 (ed. Kühn, 10:982–84).
26. "honeylike": Cf. Galen, *De methodo medendi* 14.12 (ed. Kühn, 10:985): μελικηρίς.
27. "Those [abscesses] whose contents resemble meal boiled in water": Cf. Galen, *De methodo medendi* 14.12 (ed. Kühn, 10:985): ἀθέρωμα.
28. "Fat-like [abscesses]": Cf. Galen, *De methodo medendi* 14.12 (ed. Kühn, 10:985): στεάτωμα.
29. Galen, *De methodo medendi* 14.12 (ed. Kühn, 10:985).
30. Cf. Galen, *De methodo medendi* 14.13 (ed. Kühn, 10:989): πτερύγια (cf. Liddell-Scott, *Greek-English Lexicon*, 1547, s.v. πτερύγιον: "disease of the eye when a membrane grows over it from the inner corner"; Ullmann, *Wörterbuch zu den griechisch-arabischen*, 569).
31. Galen, *De methodo medendi* 14.13 (ed. Kühn, 10:988–89).
32. I.e., that of curing the patient.
33. Cf. Maimonides, *On Asthma* 13.17–19 (ed. and trans. Bos, 1:89–91).
34. Galen, *De methodo medendi* 14.13 (ed. Kühn, 10:989).
35. I.e., varicose.
36. I.e., polyps.
37. "and, in some cases, together with the entire nose": Not in Galen.
38. Galen, *De methodo medendi* 14.13 (ed. Kühn, 10:988).
39. "pterygium": I.e., a winglike membrane growing over the eye from the inner corner (see aphorism 15.21 above); cf. Galen, *De methodo medendi* 14.19 (ed. Kühn, 10:989).
40. Galen, *De methodo medendi* 14.19 (ed. Kühn, 10:1018).
41. "[chalazion]": Cf. Galen, *De methodo medendi* 14.19 (ed. Kühn, 10:1019): χαλάζιον.
42. *kumna*: "hidden [matter]." The formation of pus behind the cornea; cf. Galen, *De methodo medendi* 14.19 (ed. Kühn, 10:1019).
43. Galen, *De methodo medendi* 14.19 (ed. Kühn, 10:1019–20).
44. "illnesses associated with pain": Galen, *De compositione medicamentorum per genera* 7.9 (ed. Kühn, 13:994), speaks about "painful inflammations."
45. Galen, *De compositione medicamentorum per genera* 7.9 (ed. Kühn, 13:994).
46. Galen, *De compositione medicamentorum secundum locos* 6.8 (ed. Kühn, 12:981–82).
47. Galen, *De methodo medendi* 13.22 (ed. Kühn, 10:935–36).
48. Galen, *De compositione medicamentorum secundum locos* 5.2 (ed. Kühn, 12:820).
49. For the couching needle (*miqdaḥ*), a broad, spatula-ended needle, see Albucasis, *On Surgery and Instruments*, ed. and trans. Lewis and Spink, 252.

50. Galen, *In Hippocratis De officina medici commentarius* 1.6 (ed. Kühn 18B:672); cf. the close parallel in Ibn Riḍwān, *Compendium of Galen's Commentary*, 104: "For after the moisture has been drained down from the eye, the couching needle must be held firmly in the place to be cleared for a considerable length of time"; see as well ʿAlī ibn ʿIsā, *Erinnerungsbuch für Augenärzte*, 120 (reprint, p. 686): "Siehst du nun, dass der Star bereits herabgestiegen, und die Pupille frei geworden, und der Star bereits an der Ort der [Traubenhaut-] Wimpern gelangt ist, dann halte eine längere Zeit hindurch die Nadel fest [und unbeweglich], bis die Wimpern, welche an der Innenfläche der Traubenhaut sitzen, den Star annehmen [ansaugen und festhalten]: danach erst hebe die Nadel empor von dem Star."

51. Galen, *De usu partium* 10.5 (ed. Helmreich, 2:71).

52. Galen, *De compositione medicamentorum per genera* 3.2 (ed. Kühn, 13:565, 594).

53. "until it assumes the consistency of bath sordes": I.e., oily sediment in baths. Cf. Galen, *De methodo medendi* 6.2 (ed. Kühn, 10:394): γλοιῶδες.

54. "bee glue": Cf. *Galen, De methodo medendi* 6.2 (ed. Kühn, 10:393): πρόπολις.

55. I.e., the same recipe with opopanax instead of sagapenum.

56. Galen, *De methodo medendi* 6.2 (ed. Kühn, 10:393–94).

57. Galen, *De methodo medendi* 6.3 (ed. Kühn, 10:401).

58. Galen, *In Hippocratis Aphorismos commentarius* 6.27 (ed. Kühn 18A:39–40).

59. I.e., hydrocele.

60. Cf. Galen, *De methodo medendi* 14.13 (ed. Kühn, 10:988): τῷ πάθει.

61 "a thong": Cf. Galen, *De methodo medendi* 14.13 (ed. Kühn, 10:988): ἱμαντώδης.

62. Galen, *De methodo medendi* 14.13 (ed. Kühn, 10:988).

63. Galen, *De methodo medendi* 6.4 (ed. Kühn, 10:415ff).

64. Galen, *De methodo medendi* 4.6 (ed. Kühn, 10:293).

65. "or by transferring it to a nearby site": Cf. Galen, *De methodo medendi* 5.5 (ed. Kühn, 10:327): παροχέτευσις (diversion).

66. "vinegar mixed [with water]": Cf. Galen, *De methodo medendi* 5.5 (ed. Kühn, 10:327): ὀξύκρατον.

67. Galen, *De methodo medendi* 5.5 (ed. Kühn, 10:326–28).

68. Galen, *De methodo medendi* 5.3 (ed. Kühn, 10:319).

69. Galen, *De methodo medendi* 5.4 (ed. Kühn, 10:324–25).

70. "livid": Cf. Galen, *De methodo medendi* 4.5 (ed. Kühn, 10:284): πελιδνός.

71. Galen, *De methodo medendi* 4.5 (ed. Kühn, 10:284).

72. Galen, *De methodo medendi* 4.2 (ed. Kühn, 10:238).

73. Galen, *In Hippocratis Epidemiarum* 6.2 (ed. Wenkebach and Pfaff [CMG 5.10.2.2], 94 lines 23–24; Deller translation, 534, no. 68).

74. "sinuous ulcer": Cf. Galen, *Ad Glauconem de methodo medendi* 2.10 (ed. Kühn, 11:129): κολπός. For the translation "sinuous ulcer," cf. Paulus Aegineta, *De re medica*, 4.38. Liddell and Scott, *Greek-English Lexicon*, 974, translates "fistulous ulcer which spreads under the skin"; and Ullmann, *Wörterbuch zu den griechisch-arabischen*, 357: "Fistel, Hohlgeschwür." For the Arabic term, cf.

Freytag, *Lexicon Arabico-Latinum*, 1:454, s.v. *makhba⁾*: "ulcus in carne, quo non afficitur os aut tendo" (an ulcer affecting the flesh, not the bones or tendons).

75. "lye from ashes": Cf. Galen, *Ad Glauconem de methodo medendi* 2.10 (ed. Kühn, 11:129): κονία.

76. *Qāṭir* is either any gum from a tree or, especially, dragon's blood; how it came to be identified with *mā⁾ al-ramād* (lye) I do not know.

77. "in a circular form": Lit., as if it were a cord that surrounds it.

78. Galen, *Ad Glauconem de methodo medendi* 2.10 (ed. Kühn, 11:127–30).

79. "although it never closes up": Cf. Galen, *De methodo medendi* 3.9 (ed. Kühn, 10:220): "although the ulcer will never heal."

80. Galen, *De methodo medendi* 3.9 (ed. Kühn, 10:220–21).

81. "even from the jugular veins": Galen, *De methodo medendi* 5.4 (ed. Kühn, 10:320), only speaks about a hemorrhage from the meninges of the brain. However, Paulus Aegineta, *De re medica* 4.53, refers to hemorrhages from the meninges of the brain, wounds of the neck, and even those of the jugular veins.

82. The hairs of the hare thus function as a kind of pledget that is to be replaced until the wound has healed.

83. Galen, *De methodo medendi* 5.4 (ed. Kühn, 10:320–21).

84. "something of the shape of a laurel leaf": Cf. Galen, *De methodo medendi* 13.5 (ed. Kühn, 10:886): μυρσινοειδῶς.

85. "direction": Lit., length.

86. Galen, *De methodo medendi* 13.5 (ed. Kühn, 10:886–87).

87. "homoiomerous parts": I.e., substances such as bone, flesh, and the humors, which have no naked-eye structure. They are formed from the four elements, which, however, are so mixed in them that none is individually perceptible.

88. Galen, *De arte parva* 34 (ed. Kühn, 1:396).

89. Galen, *Ad Glauconem de methodo medendi* 2.3 (ed. Kühn, 11:84) speaks about inflammations caused by a defluxion of humors: τὰς ἐπὶ τοῖς ῥεύμασιν φλεγμονὰς.

90. "*ḥumra*": I.e., erysipelas.

91. Galen, *Ad Glauconem de methodo medendi* 2.3 (ed. Kühn, 11:84).

92. "*ḥumra*": I.e., erysipelas.

93. "when its seething heat subsides": Lit., when its heat subsides and its boiling stops. Cf. Galen, *Ad Glauconem de methodo medendi* 2.3 (ed. Kühn, 11:84): ἡνίκα δ᾽ ἤδη τὸ ζέον ἄπεστιν αὐτοῦ.

94. Galen, *Ad Glauconem de methodo medendi* 2.3 (ed. Kühn, 11:84–85).

95. "cataplasm made of figs": Cf. Galen, *Ad Glauconem de methodo medendi* 2.9 (ed. Kühn, 11:119): κατάπλασμα τῶν ἡψημένων ἰσχάδων (a cataplasm made from boiled dried figs).

96. Galen, *Ad Glauconem de methodo medendi* 2.9 (ed. Kühn, 11:119–20).

97. "treatment": Galen adds "like wounds" (ὥσπερ τραύματα).

98. Galen, *Ad Glauconem de methodo medendi* 2.9 (ed. Kühn, 11:119).

99. "*ṣadīd*": Lit. rust; cf. Galen, *De methodo medendi* 3.3 (ed. Kühn, 10:176): ἰχώρ (serum, fluid, watery moisture; cf. Ullmann, *Wörterbuch zu den griechisch-arabischen*, 317).

100. *"waḍar"*: I.e., filth; cf. Galen, *De methodo medendi* 3.3 (ed. Kühn, 10:176): ῥυπαρόν; cf. Ullmann, *Wörterbuch zu den griechisch-arabischen*, 594, s.v. ῥυπαρός.

101. "the thin or the thick secretion": Lit., one of these secretions.

102. Galen, *De methodo medendi* 3.3 (ed. Kühn, 10:176).

103. According to Dietrich in Dioscurides, *Dioscurides Triumphans*, ed. Dietrich, 3.96, *sawsan* usually means the white lily.

104. "lily (*Lilium*) roots": Galen, *De methodo medendi* 3.3 (ed. Kühn, 10:177), recommends iris (ἴρις) and birthwort (ἀριστολοχία).

105. "tutty": Galen, *De methodo medendi* 3.3 (ed. Kühn, 10:177), recommends cadmia (καδμεία). Tutty was often confused with cadmia; cf. Maimonides, *Glossary of Drug Names*, ed. Rosner, no. 382.

106. "wine": Galen, *De methodo medendi* 3.3 (ed. Kühn, 10:177), recommends zinc oxide (πομφόλυξ).

107. Galen, *De methodo medendi* 3.3 (ed. Kühn, 10:177).

108. "A remedy that closes a wound with flesh": Cf. Galen, *De methodo medendi* 3.5 (ed. Kühn, 10:192): τὸ κολλητικὸν; Ullmann, *Wörterbuch zu den griechisch-arabischen*, s.v. κολλητικός.

109. "a remedy that makes the flesh grow": Cf. Galen, *De methodo medendi* 3.5 (ed. Kühn, 10:192): τὸ σαρκωτικὸν.

110. "unripe": Cf. Galen, *De methodo medendi* 3.5 (ed. Kühn, 10:199): ὀμφακίτης.

111. "Egyptian thorn": Cf. Galen, *De methodo medendi* 3.5 (ed. Kühn, 10:199): ἄκανθα Αἰγυπτία; cf. Löw, *Aramäische Pflanzennamen*, 196–97, s.v. القرظ.

112. "rose or blossom of the wild pomegranate": Cf. Dioscurides, *Dioscurides Triumphans*, ed. Dietrich, 1.82.

113. Galen, *De methodo medendi* 3.5 (ed. Kühn, 10:192, 198–99).

114. Galen, *De methodo medendi* 3.6 (ed. Kühn, 10:201–2).

115. "[as a treatment for a cold and lasting catarrh]": In Galen, *De instrumento odoratus* (ed. Kollesch, 46:3–4), Galen relates how he treated a patient whose sense of smell was impeded because of a cold and lasting catarrh; cf. al-Rāzī, *Kitāb al-ḥāwī*, 3:66.

116. Galen, *De instrumento odoratus* (ed. Kollesch, 46:3–4). For this text see Maimonides, *Medical Aphorisms* 1.41 (ed. and trans. Bos, 1:17).

117. According to Galen, *De atra bile* (ed. De Boer, 78 line 23), the eminent physician was Stratonicus, one of his teachers in Pergamum.

118. "the first day [thereafter]": I.e., the next day, which is the second day; cf. Galen, *De atra bile* (ed. De Boer, 78 lines 25–26): κατὰ τὴν ὑστεραίαν.

119. Galen, *De atra bile* (ed. De Boer, 78 lines 19–29).

120. Galen, *In Hippocratis De officina medici commentarius* 1.13 (ed. Kühn, 18B:686–87); cf. ʿAlī ibn Riḍwān, *Compendium of Galen's Commentary*, 106–7.

121. Galen, *In Hippocratis De officina medici commentarius* 2.29 (ed. Kühn, 18B:804–5); cf. ʿAlī ibn Riḍwān, *Compendium of Galen's Commentary*, 110–11.

122. "ribs": Lit., sides; cf. Galen, *In Hippocratem De alimento commentarius* 4.22 (ed. Kühn, 15:409): πλευραί. The term features only in the Hippocratic text and not in Galen's commentary, which is a Renaissance forgery.

123. "upper arm": Cf. Galen, *In Hippocratem De alimento commentarius* 4.22 (ed. Kühn, 15:409): πῆχυς (forearm).

124. "forearm": Cf. Galen, *In Hippocratem De alimento commentarius* 4.22 (ed. Kühn, 15:409): βραχίων (upper arm).

125. Galen, *In Hippocratem De alimento commentarius* 4.22 (ed. Kühn, 15:409).

126. For this commentary by Asklepios, which is unknown from bibliographical literature, see the introduction to this volume (pp. xiii–xiv).

127. "broken bones": Galen, *De methodo medendi* 6.5 (ed. Kühn, 10:441), speaks about multiple fractures, especially with ulcers.

128. Galen, *De methodo medendi* 6.5 (ed. Kühn, 10:441).

129. Galen, *In Hippocratis De officina medici commentarius* 3.33 (ed. Kühn, 18B:895–96); cf. ʿAlī ibn Riḍwān, *Compendium of Galen's Commentary*, 118–21.

130. Galen, *In Hippocratis De officina medici commentarius* 3.21 (ed. Kühn, 18B:862); cf. ʿAlī ibn Riḍwān, *Compendium of Galen's Commentary*, 116–17.

131. "cast": Cf. ʿAlī ibn Riḍwān, *Compendium of Galen's Commentary*, 117 line 14: "box splint."

132. Galen, *In Hippocratis De officina medici commentarius* 3.19 (ed. Kühn, 18B:850); cf. ʿAlī ibn Riḍwān, *Compendium of Galen's Commentary*, 116–17.

133. Galen, *In Hippocratis De officina medici commentarius* 3.4, 12 (ed. Kühn, 18B:825, 832); cf. ʿAlī ibn Riḍwān, *Compendium of Galen's Commentary*, 112–15.

134. "three": Cf. Galen, *In Hippocratis De officina medici commentarius* 3.2 (ed. Kühn, 18B:821): "three or four."

135. Galen, *In Hippocratis De officina medici commentarius* 3.2 (ed. Kühn, 18B:821); cf. ʿAlī ibn Riḍwān, *Compendium of Galen's Commentary*, 112–13.

Bibliographies

Translations and Editions of Works by
or Attributed to Moses Maimonides
(arranged alphabetically by translator or editor)

Bos, Gerrit, ed. and trans. *On Asthma*. Provo, Utah: Brigham Young University Press, 2002.
———, ed. and trans. *Medical Aphorisms: Treatises 1–5*. Provo, Utah: Brigham Young University Press, 2004.
———, ed. and trans. *Medical Aphorisms: Treatises 6–9*. Provo, Utah: Brigham Young University Press, 2007.
Bos, Gerrit, and Michael R. McVaugh, ed. and trans. *On Asthma. Volume 2*. Provo, Utah: Brigham Young University Press, 2008.
———, ed. and trans. *On Poisons and the Protection against Lethal Drugs*. Provo, Utah: Brigham Young University Press, 2009.
Kahle, Paul. "Mosis Maimonidis Aphorismorum praefatio et excerpta." In *Galeni in Platonis Timaeum commentarii fragmenta*. Edited by Heinrich Otto Schröder, Appendix 2. Corpus Medicorum Graecorum, Supplement 1. Leipzig: Teubner, 1934.
Muntner, Süssman, ed. *Pirḳe Mosheh bi-refuʾah: be-targumo shel Natan ha-Meʾati*. Jerusalem: Mosad ha-Rav Ḳuḳ, 1959.
Rosner, Fred, trans. *The Medical Aphorisms of Maimonides*. Maimonides' Medical Writings 3. Haifa: Maimonides Research Institute, 1989.
———, ed. and trans. *Moses Maimonides' Glossary of Drug Names*. Maimonides' Medical Writings 7. Haifa: Maimonides Research Institute, 1995.

Editions of Galenic Works
(arranged alphabetically by translator or editor)

Alexanderson, Bengt, ed. *Peri Kriseōn* (*De crisibus*). Göteborg: Almquist & Wiksell, 1967.
Brain, Peter. *Galen on Bloodletting: A Study of the Origins, Development and Validity of His Opinions, with a Translation of the Three Works*. Cambridge: Cambridge University Press, 1986.

Deller, K. H. "Die Exzerpte des Moses Maimonides aus den Epidemienkommentaren des Galen." Supplement to Galen, *In Hippocratis Epidemiarum librum VI commentaria I–VIII.* Edited by Ernst Wenkebach and Franz Pfaff. Corpus Medicorum Graecorum 5.10.2.2. Berlin: Academia Verlag, 1956.

Green, Robert Montraville, trans. *A Translation of Galen's* Hygiene. Introduction by Henry E. Sigerist. Springfield, IL: Thomas 1951. (See also Koch's edition below.)

Helmreich, Georg, ed. *De usu partium.* 2 vols. Bibliotheca Scriptorum Graecorum et Romanorum Teubneriana. Leipzig: Teubner, 1907–9. Reprint, Amsterdam: Adolf M. Hakkert, 1968. (See also May's translation below.)

———, ed. In *Hippocratis de victu acutorum commentaria.* Corpus Medicorum Graecorum 5.9.1. Leipzig: Teubner, 1914.

Iskandar, Albert Z., ed. and trans. *On Examinations by Which the Best Physicians Are Recognized.* Corpus Medicorum Graecorum, Supplementum Orientale 4. Berlin: Akademie Verlag, 1988.

Koch, Konrad, ed. *De sanitate tuenda.* Corpus Medicorum Graecorum 5.4.2. Leipzig: Teubner, 1923. (See also Green's translation above.)

Kollesch, Jutta, ed. and trans. *De instrumento odoratus.* Corpus Medicorum Graecorum 5. Berlin: Akademie, 1964.

Kühn, Karl Gottlob, ed. *Claudii Galeni opera omnia.* 20 vols. 1821–33. Reprint, Hildesheim, Germany: Georg Olms, 1964–67.

May, Margaret Tallmadge, trans. *Galen on the Usefulness of the Parts of the Body.* 2 vols. Ithaca, NY: Cornell University Press, 1968. (See also Helmreich's edition above.)

Mewaldt, Johannes, ed. *In Hippocratis De natura hominis commentaria tria.* Corpus Medicorum Graecorum 5.9.1. Leipzig: Teubner, 1914.

Siegel, Rudolph E., trans. *Galen on the Affected Parts.* New York: Karger, 1976.

Stern, S. M., ed. and trans. "Maimonides' *Treatise to a Prince, Containing Advice on Sexual Matters.*" In *Maimonidis Commentarius in Mischnam: E codicibus Hunt. 117 et Pococke 295 in Bibliotheca Bodleiana Oxoniensi servatis et 72–73 bibliothecae Sassooniensis Letchworth.* Edited by S. M. Stern, 17–21. Corpus codicum Hebraicorum Medii Aevi 1.3. Copenhagen: Ejnar Munksgaard, 1966.

Wasserstein, Abraham, ed. and trans. *Galen's Commentary on the Hippocratic Treatise "Airs, Waters, Places": in the Hebrew Translation of Solomon ha-Me'ati.* Proceedings of the Israel Academy of Sciences and Humanities 6.3. Jerusalem: Israel Academy of Sciences and Humanities, 1983.

Wenkebach, Ernst, and Franz Pfaff, ed. *Galeni in Hippocratis Epidemiarum librum I–III commentaria V.* In *Hippocratis Epidemiarum commentaria I–VIII, Indices.* Corpus Medicorum Graecorum 5.10.1, 5.10.2.1, 5.10.2.2, 5.10.2.4. Leipzig and Berlin: Teubner-Akademie Verlag, 1934–56.

General Bibliography

Álvarez-Millán, Cristina. "Actualización del corpus médico-literario de los Banū Zuhr: Nota bibliográfica." *Al-qanṭara: Revista de estudios árabes* 16, no. 1 (1995): 173–80.

Anastassiou, Anargyros, and Dieter Irmer, ed. *Testimonien zum Corpus Hippocraticum.* Part 2, *Galen.* Vol. 1, *Hippokrateszitate in den Kommentaren und im Glossar.* Göttingen, Germany: Vandenhoeck and Ruprecht, 1997.

Aristotle. *Aristotle's "De anima" Translated into Hebrew by Zeraḥyah ben Isaac ben Sheʾaltiel Ḥen: A Critical Edition with an Introduction and Index.* Edited by Gerrit Bos. Leiden: Brill, 1994.

Baron, Salo Wittmeyer. *A Social and Religious History of the Jews.* Vol. 8, *High Middle Ages, 500–1200: Philosophy and Science.* 2nd edition, revised and enlarged. New York: Columbia University Press, 1952–92.

Beit-Arié, Malachi, comp., and R. A. May, ed. *Catalogue of the Hebrew Manuscripts in the Bodleian Library: Supplement of Addenda and Corrigenda to Vol. 1 (A. Neubauer's Catalogue).* Oxford: Clarendon, 1994. (See also Neubauer's catalogue below.)

Blau, Joshua. *The Emergence and Linguistic Background of Judaeo-Arabic: A Study of the Origins of Middle Arabic.* Jerusalem: Ben Zvi Institute, 1981.

Bos, Gerrit. "Maimonides' Medical Works and their Contribution to his Medical Biography." *Maimonidean Studies* 5 (2008): 243–66.

Cano Ledesma, Aurora. *Indización de los manuscritos árabes de El Escorial.* Madrid: Ediciones Escurialenses, Real Biblioteca de El Escorial, 1996.

Deichgräber, Karl. *Hippokrates' De humoribus in der Geschichte der griechischen Medizin.* Abhandlungen der Geistes- und sozialwissenschaftlichen Klasse, vol. 1972, no. 14. Mainz: Akademie der Wissenschaften und der Literatur, 1972.

Derenbourg, Hartwig, comp., and Henri Paul Joseph Renaud, ed. *Médecine et histoire naturelle.* Vol. 2, fasc. 2 of *Les manuscrits arabes de l'Escurial.* Publications de l'Ecole nationale des langues orientales vivantes. Paris: LeRoux, 1939.

Dioscurides. *Dioscurides triumphans: Ein anonymer arabischer Kommentar (Ende 12. Jahrh. n. Chr.) zur "Materia medica."* Edited and translated by Albert Dietrich. 2 vols. Göttingen: Vandenhoeck and Ruprecht, 1988.

Dozy, Reinhart Pieter Anne. *Supplément aux dictionnaires arabes.* 2nd ed. 2 vols. Leiden: Brill, 1927.

Freudenthal, Gad. "Les sciences dans les communautés juives médiévales de Provence: leur appropriation, leur rôle." *Revue des études juives,* vol. 152, fasc. 1–2 (1993): 29–136.

Freytag, Georg Wilhelm. *Lexicon Arabico-Latinum.* 4 vols. Halle, Germany: Schwetschke and Son, 1830–37.

Gross, Henri. *Gallia Judaica: Dictionnaire géographique de la France d'après les sources rabbiniques. Traduit sur le manuscript de l'auteur par Moïse Bloch.* Paris: Librairie Léopold Cerf, 1897.

Hinz, Walther. *Islamische Masse und Gewichte: Umgerechnet ins metrische System.* Handbuch der Orientalistik 1, Ergänzungs-band 1.1. 1955. Photomechanical reprint, Leiden: Brill, 1970.

Hippocrates. *Oeuvres complètes d'Hippocrate.* Translated by É. Littré. 10 vols. 1839–61. Reprint, Amsterdam: Hackert, 1973–89.

———. *Regimen.* In *Hippocrates.* Translated by William Henry Samuel Jones. Loeb Classical Library 147–50. 1923–31. Reprint, Cambridge, MA: Harvard University Press, 1979.

Hopkins, S. "The Languages of Maimonides." In *The Trias of Maimonides: Jewish, Arabic, and Ancient Culture of Knowledge* (Die Trias des Maimonides: Jüdische, arabische, und antike Wissenskultur). Edited by Georges Tamer, 85–106. Studia Judaica 30. New York: de Gruyter, 2005.

Ibn ʿAbbās al-Zahrāwī, Abū al-Qāsim Khalaf (Albucasis). *Albucasis: On Surgery and Instruments: A Definitive Edition of the Arabic Text with English Translation and Commentary.* Edited and translated by Geoffrey L. Lewis and Martin S. Spink. London: The Wellcome Institute of the History of Medicine, 1973.

Ibn Abī Uṣaybiʿa. *ʿUyūn al-anbāʾ fī ṭabaqāt al-aṭibbāʾ.* Beirut: Dār Maktabat al-Ḥayāt, n.d.

Ibn al-ʿAbbās al-Mājūsī, Alī. *Kāmil al-Ṣināʿa al-ṭibbīya,* 2 vols. Egypt: Būlāq, 1877.

Ibn al-Nadīm. *Kitab al-Fihrist.* Cairo: Miṭbaʿa al-istiqāma, 1928.

———. *Mani, siene Lehre und seine Schriften; ein Beitrag zur Geschichte des Manichäismus.* Edited by Gustav Flügel. Leipzig: Brockhaus, 1862.

Ibn ʿIsā al-Kaḥḥāl, ʿAlī. *Erinnerungsbuch für Augenärzte: Aus arabischen Handschriften.* Translated by J. Hirschberg und J. Lippert. Leipzig: Verlag von Veit, 1904. Reprint, 1996: *Augenheilkunde im Islam: Texte, Studien und Übersetzungen.* Vol. 1. Edited by Fuat Sezgin. Veröffentlichungen des Institutes für Geschichte der Arabisch-Islamischen Wissenschaften 44. Reihe B: Nachdrucke, Abt. Medizin. Band 3.1.

Ibn Riḍwān, ʿAlī. *Compendium of Galen's Commentary on Hippocrates' KAT' IHTREION.* Edited and translated by M. Lyons. Corpus Medicorum Graecorum, Supplementum Orientale I. Berlin: Akademie Verlag, 1963.

Ibn Sahl, Sābūr. *Dispensatorium parvum (al-aqrābādhin al-ṣaghīr).* Edited by Oliver Kahl. Islamic Philosophy, Theology, and Science: Texts and Studies 16. Leiden: Brill, 1994.

Kaufmann, David. "Le neveu de Maïmonide." *Revue des études juives* 7 (1883): 152–53.

Koningsveld, P. Sj. van. "Andalusian-Arabic Manuscripts from Christian Spain: A Comparative, Intercultural Approach." *Israel Oriental Studies* 12 (1992): 75–110.

Kraemer, Joel L. *Maimonides: The Life and World of One of Civilization's Greatest Minds.* New York: Doubleday, 2008.

———. "Six Unpublished Maimonides Letters from the Cairo Genizah." In *Maimonidean Studies* 2. Edited by A. Hyman, 61–94. New York: Yeshiva University Press, 1991.

Lane, Edward William. *Arabic-English Lexicon.* London: Williams and Norgate, 1863–79.

Langermann, Y. Tzvi. "Arabic Writings in Hebrew Manuscripts: A Preliminary Listing." *Arabic Sciences and Philosophy* 6, no. 1 (March 1996): 137–60.

――――. "Maimonides on the Synochous Fever." *Israel Oriental Studies* 13 (1993): 175–98.

Leclerc, Lucien. *Histoire de la médecine arabe*. 2 vols. Paris: Leroux, 1876.

Liddell, H. G., and R. Scott. *A Greek-English Lexicon*. Revised and augmented throughout by H. S. Jones a.o. With a supplement 1968. Reprint, Oxford: Clarendon Press, 1989.

Löw, Immanuel. *Aramäische Pflanzennamen*. Leipzig: Engelmann, 1881.

Meyerhof, Max. "The Medical Work of Maimonides." In *Essays on Maimonides: An Octocentennial Volume*. Edited by Salo Wittmayer Baron, 265–99. New York: Columbia University Press, 1941.

――――. "Über echte und unechte Schriften Galens, nach arabischen Quellen." *Sitzungsberichte der Preussischen Akademie der Wissenschaften: Philosophisch-historische Klasse* 28 (1928): 533–48.

Neubauer, Adolf. *Catalogue of the Hebrew Manuscripts in the Bodleian Library and in the College Libraries of Oxford*. 1886–1906. Reprint, Oxford: Clarendon, 1994. (See also Beit-Arié's supplement above.)

Oribasius. *Collectiones Medicae*. Edited by Johann Raeder. Corpus Medicorum Graecorum 6.1–2. 4 vols. Leipzig: Teubner, 1928–33.

Paulus Aegineta. *De re medica*. Edited by J. L. Heiberg. Corpus Medicorum Graecorum 9. 2 vols. Leipzig: Teubner, 1921–24.

Pertsch, Wilhelm. *Die arabischen Handschriften der herzoglichen Bibliothek zu Gotha*. Vol. 4, pt. 3, *Die Orientalischen Handschriften der herzoglichen Bibliothek zu Gotha*. Gotha, Germany: Perthes, 1877–92.

Ravitzky, Aviezer. "Mishnato shel R. Zeraḥyah ben Isaac ben Sheʾaltiel Ḥen." PhD diss., Hebrew University, 1977.

Rāzī, Abū Bakr Muḥammad ben Zakarīyāʾ al-. *Kitāb al-ḥāwī fī al ṭibb*. Vols. 1–23. Hyderabad: Daʾiratu al-Maʿarifʾl-Osmania (Osmania Oriental Publications Bureau), Osmania University, 1952–74.

Richter-Bernburg, Lutz, trans. "Eine arabische Version der pseudogalenischen Schrift *De Theriaca ad Pisonem*." PhD diss., University of Göttingen, 1969.

Schacht, Joseph, and Max Meyerhof. "Maimonides against Galen, on Philosophy and Cosmogony." *Bulletin of the Faculty of Arts of the University of Egypt* 5, no. 1 (1937): 53–88 (Arabic Section).

Sezgin, Fuat. *Geschichte des arabischen Schrifttums*. Vol. 3, *Medizin-Pharmazie-Zoologie-Tierheilkunde bis ca. 430 H*. Leiden: Brill, 1970.

Sirat, Colette. "Une liste de manuscrits du Dalālat al-ḥayryn." *Maimonidean Studies* 4 (2000): 109–33.

Steinschneider, Moritz. *Die arabischen Übersetzungen aus dem Griechischen*. 1889–96. Reprint, Graz, Austria: Akademische Druck- und Verlagsanstalt, 1960.

――――. "Die griechischen Ärzte in arabischen Übersetzungen." *Virchows Archiv* 124 (1891): 115–36, 268–96, 455–87.

――――. *Die hebräischen Handschriften der K. Hof- und Staatsbibliothek in München*. 2nd ed. Munich: Palm'sche Hofbuchhandlung, 1895.

――――. *Die hebräischen Übersetzungen des Mittelalters und die Juden als Dolmetscher*. 1893. Reprint, Graz, Austria: Akademische Druck- und Verlagsanstalt, 1956.

———. "Eine altfranzösische Compilation eines Juden über die Fieber." *Virchow's Archiv* 136 (1894): 399–402.

———. *Verzeichniss der hebräischen Handschriften in Berlin.* 2 vols. 1878–97. Reprint, in 1 vol., Hildesheim, Germany: Olms, 1980.

Tamīmī, Muḥammad ibn Aḥmad al-. *Über die Steine: Das 14. Kapitel aus dem "Kitāb al-Muršid" des Muḥammad ibn Aḥmad at-Tamīmī, nach dem Pariser Manuskript.* Edited and translated by Jutta Schönfeld. Islamkundliche Untersuchungen 38. Freiburg: Schwarz, 1976.

Thies, Hans-Jürgen. *Erkrankungen des Gehirns insbesondere Kopfschmerzen in der arabischen Medizin.* Beiträge zur Sprach- und Kulturgeschichte des Orients 19. Walldorf, Hessen, Germany: Verlag für Orientkunde, 1968.

Ullmann, Manfred. *Die Medizin im Islam.* Handbuch der Orientalistik 1, Ergänzungsband 6.1. Leiden: Brill, 1970.

———. *Islamic medicine.* Translated by Jean Watt. Edinburgh: Edinburgh University Press, 1978.

———. *Wörterbuch zu den griechisch-arabischen Übersetzungen des 9. Jahrhunderts.* Wiesbaden: Harrassowitz, 2002.

———. *Wörterbuch zu den griechisch-arabischen Übersetzungen des 9. Jahrhunderts.* Supplement. Vol. 1: A–O. Wiesbaden: Harrassowitz, 2006.

———. *Wörterbuch zu den griechisch-arabischen Übersetzungen des 9. Jahrhunderts.* Supplement. Vol. 2: Pi–Omega. Wiesbaden: Harrassowitz, 2007.

———. "Zwei spätantike Kommentare zu der hippokratischen Schrift 'De morbis muliebribus.'" *Medizinhistorisches Journal* 12 (1977): 245–62.

Vajda, Georges. *Index général des manuscrits arabes musulmans de la Bibliothèque nationale de Paris.* Publication de l'Institut de recherche et d'histoire des textes 4. Paris: Éditions du Centre national de la recherche scientifique, 1953.

Vogelstein, Hermann, and Paul Rieger. *Geschichte der Juden in Rom.* 2 vols. Berlin: Mayer and Müller, 1895–96.

Voorhoeve, Petrus, comp. *Handlist of Arabic Manuscripts in the Library of the University of Leiden and Other Collections in the Netherlands.* 2nd ed. The Hague: Leiden University Press, 1980.

Zonta, Mauro. "A Hebrew Translation of Hippocrates' De superfoetatione: Historical Introduction and Critical Edition." *Aleph: Historical Studies in Science and Judaism* 3 (2003): 97–143.

Zotenberg, Hermann, ed. *Manuscrits orientaux: Catalogues des manuscrits hébreux et samaritains de la Bibliothèque impériale.* Paris: Imprimerie impériale, 1866.

Index of Subjects

Explanatory Note: The entries are indexed by chapter and paragraph numbers. The digit 0 refers to the chapter introduction; its use indicates that the entire chapter deals with the subject.

Addenda and Corrigenda
to *Medical Aphorisms*
Volumes 1 and 2

Medical Aphorisms: Treatises 1–5

Arabic text:

Introduction (p. 3 line 11): أعرف. Read أعرِف.

1.64 (p. 23 line 7): اورمساواة[و]. Read مساواة.

2.8 (p. 28 line 10–18—p. 29 line 2): The Hebrew text quoted is that by Zerahyah, MS Munich 111.

3.52 (p. 46, footnote to line 5): للعصابع Read الأصابع.

English translation:

Introduction (p. 3 line 18): "I know." *Read* "I make it known."

1.10 (p. 9 line 15): "Most of them." *Read* "Most ligaments."

3.6 (p. 35 line 13): "Porous bodies which are porous."
Read "Porous bodies."

Medical Aphorisms: Treatises 6–9

Translator's Introduction:

p. xxiv: "Escorial, Real Biblioteca de El Escorial 869 (**S**)."
Read "Escorial, Real Biblioteca de El Escorial 869 (**Es**)."
Cf. sigla on p. xi.

"Oxford, Bodleian, Uri 412, Poc. 319, cat. Neubauer 2113 (**B**)."
Read "Oxford, Bodleian, Uri 412, Poc. 319, cat. Neubauer 2113 (**O**)."
Cf. sigla on p. xi.

p. xxv: "Oxford, Bodleian, Hunt. Donat 33, Uri 423, cat. Neubauer
2114 (**O**)." *Read* "Oxford, Bodleian, Hunt. Donat 33, Uri 423, cat.
Neubauer 2114 (**Ox**)." Cf. sigla on p. xi.

Arabic text:

6.7 (p. 2 line 15): حسّ. Read جنس.

6.10 (p. 3 line 13): بجير. Read بخير.

7.8 (p. 25 line 17): إن أهمل. Read أن أهمل.

7.61 (p. 39 line 5): إن قوما. Read أن قوما.

8.17 (p. 46 line 1): إلى الصدر. Read إلى الصدر والمعدة.

8.47 (p. 52 line 2): وحده. Read وحدّة.

9.43 (p. 68 line 8): مسرع. Add variant reading to critical apparatus:
مصرع **L**.

9.62 (p. 72, critical apparatus): ١١٤. أوائل. Read ١٤. أوائل.

9.104 (p. 81 line 14): باردا. Read بار زا.

9.109 (p. 83, critical apparatus to line 1): جمتها. Read حمّتها.

9.116 (p. 84 line 6): وأتى أمرك. Read وإنّي أمرك. Critical apparatus to the
same line: وأتى أمرك. Read وإنّي أمرك.

9.123: منقالان. Read مثقالان.

English translation:

6.7 (p. 2 lines 24–25): "a sensation of." *Read* "a kind of."

7.60 (p. 39 line 2): "*In Hippocratis Epidemiarum* 6.8." *Read* "*In Hippocratis
Epidemiarum* 6.6."

7.61 (p. 39 lines 6–7): "to weaken and extinguish the animal faculty.
Some." *Read* "to weaken and extinguish the animal faculty [to a
degree] that."

8.17 (p. 46 line 2): "to the chest." *Read* "to the chest and stomach."

8.47 (p. 52 line 4): "with a medication that has only a heating effect."
Read "with a hot and sharp medication."

9.104 (p. 81 line 25): "when the affected organ is evidently cold."
   Read "when the affected organ is external and visible."

9.104 (p. 81 lines 29–30): "When the part is markedly cold."
   Read "When the external organ is cold."

9.110 (p. 83 lines 19–20): "both young and old." *Read* "in young people and in those who were past their prime."

9.116 (p. 84 line 10): "And finally one should thicken." *Read* "And I advise you to thicken."

About the Editor / Translator

GERRIT BOS, chair of the Martin Buber Institute for Jewish Studies at the University of Cologne, was born in the Netherlands and educated both there and in Jerusalem and London. He is proficient in classical and Semitic languages, as well as in Jewish and Islamic studies. He has been research assistant at the Free University in Amsterdam, a research fellow and lecturer at University College in London, a tutor in Jewish studies at Leo Baeck College in London, and a Wellcome Institute research fellow. He currently resides in Germany with his wife and three children.

Professor Bos is widely published in the fields of Jewish studies, Islamic studies, Judeo-Arabic texts, and medieval Islamic science and medicine, having many books and articles to his credit. In addition to preparing The Medical Works of Moses Maimonides, Professor Bos is also involved with a series of medical-botanical Arabic-Hebrew-Romance synonym texts written in Hebrew characters, an edition of Ibn al-Jazzār's *Zād al-musāfir* (Viaticum), and an edition of Averroës' commentary on the zoological works of Aristotle, extant only in Hebrew and Latin translations. He received the Maurice Amado award for his work on Maimonides' medical texts.

A Note on the Types

The English text of this book was set in BASKERVILLE, a typeface originally designed by John Baskerville (1706–1775), a British stonecutter, letter designer, typefounder, and printer. The Baskerville type is considered to be one of the first "transitional" faces—a deliberate move away from the "old style" of the Continental humanist printer. Its rounded letterforms presented a greater differentiation of thick and thin strokes, the serifs on the lowercase letters were more nearly horizontal, and the stress was nearer the vertical—all of which would later influence the "modern" style undertaken by Bodoni and Didot in the 1790s. Because of its high readability, particularly in long texts, the type was subsequently copied by all major typefoundries. (The original punches and matrices still survive today at Cambridge University Press.) This adaptation, designed by the Compugraphic Corporation in the 1960s, is a notable departure from other versions of the Baskerville typeface by its overall typographic evenness and lightness in color. To enhance its range, supplemental diacritics and ligatures were created in 1997 for exclusive use in this series.

The Arabic text was set in NASKH, designed by Thomas Milo (b. 1950), a pioneer of Arabic script research, typeface design, and smart font technology in the digital era. The Naskh calligraphic style arose in Baghdad during the tenth century and became very widespread and refined during the Ottoman period. It has been favored ever since for its clarity, elegance, and versatility. Milo designed and expanded this typeface during 1992–1995 at the request of Microsoft's Middle East Product Development Department and extended its typographic range even further in subsequent editions. Milo's designs pushed the existing typographic possibilities to their limits and led to the creation of a new generation of Arabic typefaces that allowed for a more authentic treatment of the script than had been possible since the advent of moveable type for Arabic.

BOOK DESIGN BY JONATHAN SALTZMAN

◆